616
Barn... ...ristiaan
...fe/Good death.

B25

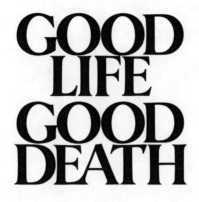

GOOD LIFE GOOD DEATH

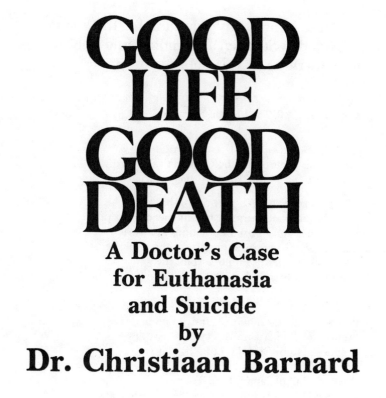

GOOD LIFE GOOD DEATH

**A Doctor's Case
for Euthanasia
and Suicide
by**

Dr. Christiaan Barnard

Prentice-Hall, Inc. Englewood Cliffs, N.J.

I wish to express my gratitude for the assistance provided by Stephen T. Donohue and Bob Molloy in the writing of this book.

Pages 50–51:
Copyright 1980, *The Houston Post,* reprinted by permission.

Good Life/Good Death: A Doctor's Case for
Euthanasia and Suicide, by Christiaan Barnard
Copyright © 1980 by Dr. Christiaan Barnard

Printed in the United States of America

Prentice-Hall International, Inc., London
Prentice-Hall of Australia, Pty. Ltd., Sydney
Prentice-Hall of Canada, Ltd., Toronto
Prentice-Hall of India Private Ltd., New Delhi
Prentice-Hall of Japan, Inc., Tokyo
Prentice-Hall of Southeast Asia Pte. Ltd., Singapore
Whitehall Books Limited, Wellington, New Zealand

10 9 8 7 6 5 4 3 2 1

Library of Congress Cataloging in Publication Data

Barnard, Christiaan Neethling.
    Good life/good death.

        Includes index.
        1. Euthanasia.   2. Right to die.   3. Suicide.
I. Title [DNLM: 1. Death.   2. Euthanasia.
3. Suicide.   4. Ethics, Medical.   W50 B259g]
R726.B27   174'.24   80-18839
ISBN 0-13-360370-9

——Contents——

Introduction

Fools have been rushing into situations since angels first showed caution. I make no apology for joining that company, though in putting down my views on life and its final end, I can hardly, in these closing years of my career as a doctor, be accused of rushing.

The question of life and its quality has long occupied my thoughts. Of death or what may lie beyond I have nothing to say. My concern is with life, the living, and improvement of the quality of our dying.

All of us die. You who read this and I who write it. Death is life's only certainty, whether it comes sooner or later, slowly or in the wink of an eye. It is a situation that faces us all and makes us one with all mankind in our mortality.

Even if we have repressed the memory, each of us can recall the moment when mortality first made itself known—perhaps an instant in childhood when it became suddenly clear that life was not forever.

I remember it as a feathery chill, like a brush of bird wings across my face, a sudden feeling of loss when told that my baby brother had died. I suppose from that moment death sprang into focus, a concrete reality that was a distinct part of being alive. And possibly it was then, at the instant of realization that life was finite, that my childhood ended.

My next strongest intimation of mortality came

when I was a thirty-five-year-old surgeon working in an American hospital. A painful ankle sent me looking for medical help, only to hear a confident American specialist diagnose my problem as rheumatoid arthritis. In a flash I was back in my fourth-year student days, ten years earlier, staring at my first patient—a little old lady crippled by the same disease.

It was then that I first paid serious attention to the question of what makes a good life and had a glimpse of the viewpoint of those who reject the thought of living anything less. For me, at that moment, all I wanted was to be a good surgeon. Accepting anything less was unthinkable.

I started work in heart surgery in the days when a large hospital department would do five open-heart operations in a week—and lose all of them. Today, the case load for a large cardiac surgery department would be many times that, and the surgeon could expect, and get, close to 100 percent success.

My career has spanned an era of great strides in medical knowledge, from the days when we felt we had done our utmost in merely diagnosing a heart condition to the point where we can now do something constructive about most, if not all, heart problems.

Yet I do not subscribe to the view that the aim of every doctor should be to conquer death. What is more relevant is to look at the problem in a slightly different way and recognize that from the instant of conception in the womb we are all dying.

This is a useful concept inasmuch as it defines one of the aims of the doctor—that is, to retard the rate of dying. But to suggest that this is the most important or even the only aim is to disregard the most vital aim of all—to ensure the patient's capacity to live to the fullest extent of his abilities.

And by living I do not mean simply exhibiting one or two vital signs, such as respiration or the registration of heartbeat. I mean rather the whole conglomeration of sensual experiences that the patient calls "being alive"—the experiences that by their very complexity and subtlety are not amenable to measurement or statistical analysis and are usually known only to the patient, his closest associates, and his doctor.

Life looked at in this way is to me so valuable that I doubt if one can set a minimum time limit on it. There is no question that modern medicine has a great deal to offer both in terms of increasing life expectancy and improving the quality of life.

In the years since I first registered at the University of Cape Town Medical School as an awed student, medical research has pushed death back beyond a number of frontiers. Some people fear that in doing so it has created a Frankenstein, a scientific caricature of the art of medicine.

That view is not mine, though at times it is tempting to adopt such a radical stand. Few reasonable people will disagree with the proposition that the civilized world would be the poorer were it not for the scientific method of continual inquiry into the physical universe.

Any attempt to put a brake on the acquisition of knowledge would, if successful, be disastrous. For not only would this deprive mankind of the fundamental right to enjoy the pride of cultural achievement, it would also retard, as surely as did Lysenkoism in Russia, the application of any possible good that could come from this knowledge.

Scientific achievement must therefore be encouraged and supported, the only requirement being that its methods conform to acceptable ethical standards.

Technological advances, on the other hand, should constantly be reviewed with the utmost vigilance. We must make sure that what is done in the name of progress is really to the good of mankind rather than to our detriment.

I do not believe it is beyond our capabilities to safeguard the future against rampant technology, at the same time deriving maximum benefit from the application of knowledge. This will require constant reexamination of our attitudes and our abilities to cope with new knowledge and new situations as they arise.

There is a French maxim which, broadly translated, says it is only the permanent that lasts. In that apparent tautology is an element of truth—for it is only by the process of adaptive change that things of permanence endure.

It is important to define the things of permanent value that we feel are worth preserving, and it is important that we adapt and change in such a way as to ensure that they remain sacred.

In this context, I believe that it is time to rethink many of our attitudes toward death and dying. We should apply the logic and reasoning that help us make other decisions in life to the events that lead up to its ending.

"One thing is certain and the rest is lies," Omár

tells us in *The Rubáiyát,* referring to the fact that death is our only certainty. Why then should it not be seen as the natural and appropriate end to a satisfying existence?

And that is what I propose to examine. With an open-door approach to technical progress, with the emergence of candor in discussions of death-related subjects, with landmark changes in ethical and legal constraints to medical practice, I feel that society is ready to take a giant step toward a better understanding of the dignity of death—and the attainment of that dignity, if necessary, through euthanasia and suicide.

It is time to look at the dilemma in which medical technology has placed us—and to consider what can be done to return the human face to *homo medicus.*

Cape Town, South Africa
August 1980

One

It is a sign of the times that every possible aspect of death is now an acceptable conversational topic. In a fifteen-year period, the number of publications on death and dying has increased almost 1,000 percent. The subject is discussed not only by medical and nursing school students but also by youngsters in elementary schools, and it is a continuing topic of interest in the media.

In my youth, growing up in the puritanical culture of South Africa in the 1930s, death was regarded as no more a fit subject for discussion than the other realities of life such as love, sex, and bodily functions.

My first unsettling thoughts about death were kindled by three pictures on the living room wall of our family home. One was a photograph of my baby brother, Abraham, sitting in a chair on a velvet cushion; another was a photograph of my mother, younger in years, dressed in black and standing at the side of a new grave; and the third was a reproduction of a painting of an angel with a baby in its arms, flying toward heaven from a grave.

Privately, I often pondered over those mementos of the absent Abraham which collectively made up a shrine for the brother I had never known.

My curiosity peaked one day when I came across a box in a drawer of my father's desk. Carefully stored inside was a little brown biscuit, hardened with age, marked on one corner by teeth marks—the last food that Abraham had eaten before his death. There was also a sharpened matchstick which my father told me had been used to clean Abraham's nails when dressing his body after death.

Today, death is more commonly discussed. Robert Dastenbaum, a psychologist, has coined the term "death awareness" to describe the mounting interest in the end of life. Acceptance of death as part of life itself has generated long-running plays, well-acclaimed films, and numerous articles.

Like everyone else, I too have tried to grasp its meaning—not only for myself as a conscious entity, as an individual ego with wants and needs, but also in terms of the greater philosophical problem facing mankind as an intelligent species.

What has concerned me most as a doctor is the growing debate on clarifying the role of the medical profession in the handling of terminal illness, and the changing demands on doctors made by new technology.

Death appears in many guises. To some, exhausted.by pain or old age, or perhaps embittered by the deterioration of the quality of life, it may come as a friend. To others, it is an enemy, intrusive and unasked. Rarely does it come in terror, a thing of fear.

In my more than thirty-five years of clinical practice I have only once seen a patient who was actually afraid while dying. He was a young man who had just had a massive heart attack. His circulation had deteriorated extensively and it was clear that he was dying. Almost his last words were, "Doctor, please help me, I don't want to die."

Generally, it is only the living who fear death, not the dying.

But whether life ends with a bang or a whimper, it is a private moment. No one can share the last fears or hopes at the bedside, and no one can intercede in a confrontation that concerns only the dying and the approach of death.

Donne said that no man is an island, that everyone is a part of the main, and that every man's death diminishes us. The poet was speaking only of life and the living. Things look a bit different to the dying.

For many, it is a time when they become enmeshed in a conspiracy of silence, the truth veiled at first in medical jargon. The patient feels his body relinquishing its hold on life as the functions break down, and though looking to the doctor for an explanation, he may still be afraid to hear it.

The doctor in turn seeks to keep the patient reassured, to allay his fears without giving false hope. The doctor must assess the patient's stability—his ability to cope with such knowledge—and decide whether the truth would help or hinder him in his final hours.

Often the doctor's job is complicated by the family's insistence on knowing the truth. He is placed in a no-win situation where the living insist on knowing and, when informed, give out an atmosphere of collusion that only serves to increase the isolation of the dying.

Even when surrounded by supportive friends and loved ones it can be a lonely journey if the dying person has not developed a life philosophy that can cope when faced with his last extremity. Even for the most stable of people, there is an awareness that this is a path never personally trodden, and although many have gone before, none has laid down guidelines. The process of dying, therefore, no matter how it is managed by the family and the medical profession, still holds a large component of loneliness for those breathing the last breath of life.

The moment of death varies according to the criteria applied, and even these vary according to whether you are looking at it from a warm, humanitarian point of view or a cold, strictly scientific angle.

In legal terms, when a man dies in the street, at home, or in the hospital, he is not dead when the ambulance collects his remains from the automobile accident, when his wife finds she cannot waken him, or when the nurse on her ward rounds cannot find a pulse. He is regarded as dead when a doctor has examined him and certified the condition. In this sense, then, a person is only dead when a doctor says he is dead.

When does a doctor certify a patient dead? Death is a clinical impression just as is the diagnosis of an illness. The impression is derived from a number of signs which make up the syndrome of death. A number of tests are applied, ranging from evidence of brain activity to heartbeat and breathing.

I have often heard people mention the exceptions that seem to disprove the rule—such as the patient who had been in a coma for months or who had a completely flat electroencephalogram (EEG)— meaning no sign of brain activity—yet made a complete recovery.

Apart from treating such reports with a pinch of salt, the common error made is in assuming that the doctor diagnoses death on the presence of a single sign. This is not so, just as appendicitis is not diagnosed merely on the presence of a pain in the abdomen.

It is the presence of a number of signs that make up the syndrome of death.

After the first heart transplant, there was a need to redefine the accepted criteria for the moment of death—as we will consider later in greater detail. When confronted with the use of such an important organ as the living heart from an apparently dead body, public reaction in many parts of the world, and certainly among the less sophisticated, was one of suspicion.

For hundreds of years, the dictum of English law held that life does not end as long as breathing continues and the heart beats. But recent advances in medical science have outdated many of the old rules and guidelines.

With hindsight, we regard this concept as erroneous. We now know that the expanding lungs and beating heart are there to keep the brain alive. As the brain is the organ that determines the quality of life, the need for these functions ceases when the brain has died.

Later on we will take a look at the Hippocratic

oath to show how much medical ethics and the approach to the treatment of patients have changed.

Take the established concept that the person is dead once the heart stops beating. From a purely scientific view, the cessation of heartbeat never coincides with the moment of death. The heart either stops before the patient dies or afterwards.

In the case of the usual heart attack, where the victim "drops dead," it is usually due to blockage of an artery supplying the heart muscle. The heart stops beating, but the patient does not die immediately. First there is loss of consciousness as the flow of blood to the brain is reduced or cut off and the person collapses.

It takes three or four minutes before there is irreparable death of the brain. At that point, the patient is dead. Hence, in this particular case, death occurs after the cessation of heartbeat.

On the other hand, a patient might suffer from severe cerebral hemorrhage (bleeding) which destroys the brain. As a result of the extensive damage to the brain, there is a cessation of respiration. This, in turn, starves the heart muscle of oxygen and leads to stoppage of the heart. In this instance, the patient dies *before* the heart stops beating.

Today's sophisticated medical technology can lead to situations in which few of the rules apply. For example, it is possible to have a heart beating for many hours in a body that is dead, and conversely, a patient can be very much alive even though the heart's beat has been stopped for hours.

Some lengthy surgical procedures are carried out without heartbeat or respiratory movements. In fact, there may not even be blood in the body, the life-giving fluid being tapped out into a reservoir until needed to restart the vital functions. Such techniques, commonplace in certain surgical procedures with small children and babies, stave off brain deterioration by cooling the tissues to very low temperatures.

In short, the signs whereby the doctor diagnoses death are not dependent on cessation of heartbeat or respiration, but on brain death. The brain is the organ that determines the quality of life, and the individual dies when his brain dies.

But there are other ways of looking at death.

Culturally, a person dies with permanent loss of consciousness. The heart may beat on, breathing may continue, the blood may circulate. But the mind, the determinant of the quality of life, is gone.

Once the brain has died, there is no need for the other body organs, and they die at various intervals thereafter. Hair and nail growth, for example, appear to continue for many hours. Total death of the body is therefore by degrees.

It is the two-way process of mental stimulation and response that makes man a cultural being. The terminally unconscious person may be surrounded by cultural stimulation but can make no response to it.

Looking at death in another way, we can call it the end of life. Hence "being alive" ends with the onset of dying. But what is life, and what do we mean when we say "I am so happy to be alive"?

Surely being alive is not simply a matter of respiration or the registration of heartbeat.

As I have said, I see it as the whole conglomeration of sensual experiences that we call "being alive"—experiences that by their very subtlety and complexity are not amenable to measurement or statistical analysis, but are certainly known to the patient, his loved ones, and his doctor. When positively felt, they contribute to the feeling we know as "happiness."

The composition of these experiences will vary from person to person. To a primitive tribesman, happiness may be simply a full stomach. Or it may mean status measured by the number of wives, cattle, and other possessions. To a small girl, it could be a colored bangle.

In the Western world a man may be content with a humdrum nine-to-five existence, with each day as predictable as the last. For another, joy in living may be bound up with adventure, excitement, novelty, even danger. Or a full life may be equated with the opportunity to listen to a good string quartet.

Each person has his own idea of how to live, and each will die a death as individual as his fingerprints.

Taking that concept one step further, each of us has an opinion as to when life no longer has meaning. When that point is reached, it gives cause to seriously consider a choice between life and death.

Doctors often see life become intolerable before the patient lapses into unconsciousness and the brain dies. The end of tolerance comes not only to the doctor and the patient but also to his family and friends, the people who know his requirements for being alive.

It is, therefore, not the diagnosis of death that concerns me as much as a possible means of determining when the state of "being alive" ceases.

In this context, dying can be defined as the irreversible deterioration of the quality of life that precedes the death of a particular individual.

——Two——

I find it disturbing that many families are preoccupied with the minutiae of death. They plan in detail for the event and make elaborate arrangements for the interment of the body. Funerals are planned in advance, care is taken in selecting just the right cemetery plot, and top priority is often given to the payment of burial insurance premiums—even when the breadwinner has to skimp on essentials to meet regular death benefit payments.

Much of this behavior is a form of psychological displacement, a concern with details, which will cause no anxiety and will keep the mind from dwelling on unpleasant realities.

To this end, it is acceptable, but how much more preferable would be a cultural conditioning toward the process of dying itself, as well as what happens once we are dead, something that would help people cope more positively with an event that sooner or later affects everyone.

As a doctor, I know full well how difficult this would be—requiring the revision of attitudes ingrained by centuries of ethnic, religious, and cultural practices.

Consider how almost all stages of life have rites of passage. This is most clearly seen in primitive communities where group membership is important. All living things react to change, to movement from the familiar to the unknown, and in animals and humans this can give rise to strongly fearful reactions.

The rite of passage, marking change from one stage to another, is usually a highly ritualized means of effecting the change with the least amount of psychological trauma while at the same time affirming group membership, the basis of all real security.

Birth is marked by ceremonies of rejoicing, propitiation of supernatural forces, and acceptance into the community. Each succeeding age-group has its time of emphasis, with puberty rites the most powerful and so on into adulthood and marriage.

In death, the community is not divided. The rites vary from place to place, but all have a common purpose: the visible declaration of change with the announcement of death to the community, the attempt to cope with change by means of ritualized mourning, other security rites such as burial or cremation ceremonies, and thereafter the strong support of the community for the bereaved.

Although it is true that some vestige of these strongly socializing and binding rituals remains in modern urban life, there has been a drift away from such public affirmation of age-group status. The group has less influence, individualism is stressed, and there is a tendency to intellectualize rather than internalize the security of group membership.

Death, and the fact of death, is hidden. It has become the province of specialists. The body is no longer kept at home for full family inspection, and we are reduced to less than the level of audience participation. We are merely notified when the body is ready for cremation or burial, and even then we have nothing directly to do with these important rites.

And in Western societies where the individual leads a secular life with little or no strong religious conviction, he is truly deprived of the comforting support of his peers in times of rapid change. Yet if we are to turn our faces from primitive ritual and belief, we must replace such social supports with others of at least equal power.

One way of doing this is by declaring open season on taboo subjects, such as euthanasia and suicide, by full and frank discussion, at least sketching out the problem and possible ways of approaching it.

The time for this is when you are in the best of health, not under the stress of approaching death—much in the way the average intelligent person would examine any other life problem. Yet most people would find open group discussion of their personal death more than a little disturbing, perhaps even bizarre, and would feel greatly inhibited in bringing into the open their own feelings on the subject.

Worldwide, religion has been man's response to the fact of death. It has developed as a source of consolation for the inconsolable, building theologies to explain the inexplicable and seeking to impart courage in the face of the unknown.

From primitive rites around a campfire to solemn ceremonies in costly and historic buildings, the aim is the same: a means of providing security against the time for change.

Whether it is a Bushman bravely urinating into the dark as he faces away from the campfire, or a cardinal administering the last rites of his faith, the central theme is one of man coping with a hostile universe by calling on his gods for support.

According to the scientists, nature abhors a vacuum. The same is true for the theologians and the mythologists. Wherever the unknown yawns, man has theorized, mythologized, and storified to fill the gap.

That which is unknown has a greater component of horror than even the most threatening concrete event. Better by far to sketch its outline, give it shape, and thereby evolve rules of coping. Man, as a sentient being in a nonsentient world, has great need to cope—to make order out of the chaos, to explain what looks like a cruel cosmic joke.

Religion played a strong role in my early years, probably more so for me than for many children growing up in the third decade of the century. My father, whom I saw as a living saint, was a Dutch Reformed missionary with a church in the small town of Beaufort West, which lies on the great plains of South Africa known as the Karroo.

My childhood was happy, even if it took place in what most South African whites would have seen as poor circumstances. I was raised with three brothers, two older and one younger. My parents, Maria and Adam Hendrik Barnard, had still another son, who died before the age of four, ironically from a heart defect that could have been repaired by the surgery I was trained to do in later years.

My father was an extremely religious man whose whole belief was that God would help him in any circumstance—financially, morally, and emotionally. Like other men of his deep spiritual convictions, he did not fear death.

For him, dying was God's will, and he truly believed that through death a person entered a better world, where all mortal suffering would disappear. He would no more question death as an integral part of man's existence on earth than he would question the presence of God in his church on the Sabbath.

Adam Barnard believed in counseling his sons in the same way as he believed in counseling his spiritual flock. On Sunday afternoons he would walk with me to the top of a hill overlooking the church—all the time listening to my childhood concerns and offering fatherly advice.

It was during one of these Sunday strolls that my father explained to me the meaning of death—leaving me perhaps more puzzled than ever.

The thought of death, in those early childhood days, had a mystery—a mystique—about it. And my attitude toward death, then as now, was greatly influenced by the deep faith of the rural Afrikaners.

It taught me that in times of crisis, such as a serious illness of a family member, religion played an important role. I saw that people who had faith in a higher power, those who believed in an afterlife, had it much easier than those who had no religious beliefs to support them in the face of death.

Yet, even against this background, I do not see

myself as basically a religious man. That is, I do not embrace a specific religion. But I do admire the personal discipline that religious belief instills in its adherents—particularly the demands of exacting faiths such as Roman Catholicism and Judaism.

I have no deep conviction in the existence of a personal God or in the geography of an actual heaven or hell. To that I must add, on the other hand, that I have not dismissed the possibility of life after death.

Call it upbringing, superstitious habit, or what you will, but I have never entered an operating theater to carry out major surgery without a silent prayer for help.

Faith, of course, is the great leveler. The most humble beggar can pray to his God in a moment of crisis. So can kings and shahs and state presidents.

But the last moment of life still carries the threat of loneliness. This was borne out by Vatican reports on Pope Paul VI which showed that, in his last years, the prelate worried about how he would die. He is reported to have often requested of his secretary, "Help me to die well."

To the religious, the advantage of their faith is that they feel no longer alone. It gives concrete limits to responsibility and helps the faithful to accept the things they cannot change.

If you don't have bread today then it is God's will, and He will give you bread tomorrow. With that in mind, going hungry for the day is less of an ordeal. You may not be happy with the state of affairs, but someone has things in hand and it will all work out for the best.

This holds for even the most ferociously

threatening of situations. Christian martyrs cheerfully dedicated their deaths to God, and many even sought martyrdom in His name. The thought of a happy life with God in the hereafter eased the pain and the loneliness of impending death.

I was deeply moved when, as an awed ten year old, my best friend, Mitchell Rossouw, told me that the last words his father spoke on his deathbed were "Death, where is thy sting?"

In any other context the words would have been a cliché. But when Mr. Rossouw uttered them he was calm, peaceful, and ready to meet his Maker.

I was enthralled by this account of a man who could look death in the face and dismiss it. Now, after nearly four decades of experience in the practice of medicine, I know that such contentment at the moment of death is not unusual.

It takes maturity to recognize that from the instant of conception we have programmed into our genes a predestined life expectancy which is finite and diminishes with every passing second.

We are, in fact, all dying. Some rapidly, some more slowly—nonetheless, we are headed for death.

I have learned from my life in medicine that death is not always an enemy. Often it is good medical treatment. Often it achieves what medicine cannot achieve—it stops suffering.

——Three——

Although death may be considered a private moment, we seldom have control over its intimacies. Even those final seconds are invaded. Mentally, the dying person has no say about the last lapse into unconsciousness. If experienced in full knowledge of what it means, it can be a time of supreme terror or even a moment of bliss.

Physically, approaching death may remove voluntary control over muscle and nerve systems, often giving great distress to the dying as the eyes no longer obey the will, the head lolls, breathing becomes difficult, and the person's sense of helplessness is magnified.

On some occasions, dying may not precede death. It may arrive suddenly, triggered by a massive coronary or by the ripping apart of vital organs in an accident.

Where life is snuffed out without warning, there is little need for controversy or discussion: Death replaces life in an instant and the dead are at peace. The problems are borne by those who mourn.

But in a long, drawn-out terminal illness, a period of dying precedes death. In such cases the family and the doctors often have the final say. Medical records are filled with case histories of terminally ill patients who were kept alive by artificial means long after there was any hope of recovery, and often long after consciousness had ceased.

The reasons for this are complex, as I hope to show in a later discussion, and are bound up with our religious and cultural values.

A scholarly analysis of human reaction to the process of dying has been provided by Dr. Elisabeth Kübler-Ross, a Swiss psychiatrist now living in Escondido, California. Her book, *On Death and Dying*, has become a classic in the literature, setting forth the stages a dying person passes through and providing valuable insight into the psychology of dying.

Dr. Kübler-Ross was one of the first to show that hospital staffs place death in the avoidance category and have even developed a defensive language when discussing it. Hospital patients do not die, they "expire." Individuals do not terminate their lives in the operating room, they are "lost on the table."

Outlining the stages of dying, Dr. Kübler-Ross points out that the first stage—denial—where the patient reacts by refusing to believe that it is happening, is often reinforced by the hospital staff because it protects them from becoming involved and from facing their own feelings.

The other stages of the dying process she has identified are as follows:

Rage and anger—or the "why me" stage, when the patient resents the fact that others remain healthy while he or she must die.

Bargaining—the "yes me, but" period, when death is accepted, but an attempt is made to strike bargains for more time. Dr. Kübler-Ross found that such patients mostly bargained with God, even those who had never talked about the Diety before. They promised to be good or to do something in exchange for another week or month or year of life.

Depression—the "yes, me" time, when the person mourns past losses, things not done, wrongs committed. From this, the person enters a stage of preparatory grief, "getting ready for the arrival of death." At this time the patient seeks quiet and does not want visitors. Dr. Kübler-Ross adds, "When a dying person doesn't want to see you anymore it is a sign he has finished his business with you and it is a blessing. He can let go peacefully."

Acceptance—the feeling of "my time is close now and it is all right." Dr. Kübler-Ross describes this final stage as "not a happy stage, but neither is it unhappy. It is devoid of feelings but it is not resignation. It's really a victory."

Of course, not every dying person goes through every stage in the exact sequence given, nor can the pace of the development from one to the other be fully predicted. But the Kübler-Ross concept of different stages of the dying process is a useful model for understanding the behavior of the patient.

The concern with death in the United States is paralleled in Britain and has attracted increasing attention on the Continent. Strangely, in spite of two thousand years of Christian teaching and an even older heritage of Greek philosophy, Western academics have only now accepted the value of the expression of grief as part of the healing process.

Rediscovery of once common attitudes toward death are an important part of the new death awareness movement, a response to the assembly-line specialization of modern life that, since the beginning of this century, has slowly and insidiously worked to separate the dying from the living.

A survey has shown that in 1900 two-thirds of Americans who died were under fifty years old, and most of them died at home. Today, most Americans, when they die, are over sixty-five and are usually in the care of a hospital or other institution. This large-scale removal of death from home to hospital has been generally experienced throughout the world.

Far from the acceptance of death as a familiar and expected result of life, Western man has allowed it to disappear from public view and into the care of the hospital and the undertaker. Finally, we have become a clinically sterile society that compartmentalizes its pains and its pleasures—a psychologically untenable position.

What has emerged is akin to a denial of death: a half-shamed admission of grief by the bereaved, and a belief that the sooner it is forgotten the better. This is helped by the modern tendency to cut ritual to the bare minimum—no ostentatious funeral, cremation rather than the dust-to-dust reminder of the open grave, and a stiff upper lip in public.

On the other hand, an obvious communications gap has evolved between those who die and those who mourn. Research in Canada has indicated that 80 percent of relatives preferred to have their terminally ill loved ones die in the hospital, while 80 percent of dying persons—like any threatened animal anxious to return to the lair—said they would prefer to die at home.

A long overdue revolution in approach has appeared in the hospice movement—the decision to regard the most important needs of the dying as relief from pain and closer contact with loved ones.

In place of the sterile hospital ward, the hospice concept substituted an easy homelike atmosphere devoid of rigid routine, an encouragement of visitors, and a positive view of the medieval "good death," in which the dying are surrounded by loved ones in an environment of mutual forgiveness.

The aim is to make death a positive experience both for the dying person and those who remain behind.

Hospice care can, of course, be offered at home, in a hospital, or in a special facility such as that made famous by Dr. Cecily Saunders of the Saint Christopher's Hospice in London. As long as the main object is met—that of helping the patient to lead as normal a life as the illness will allow—then the circumstances of care are largely irrelevant.

Dr. Saunders, with whom I had the privilege of debating several years ago, defines modern hospice in terms of the medieval hospices, which were places of hospitality run by religious groups who gave rest and comfort to pilgrims on their journey to the Holy Land. She sees this as symbolic of the journey the dying take on their way from this life to the next. The concept is given form in the statue of Saint Christopher, the patron saint of travelers, that greets visitors to her London facility.

As I indicated in the introduction to this book, the time has come to do something about the dilemma in which medical technology has placed us.

Another British authority on problems of caring for the terminally ill, Dr. Robert G. Twycross, says that the hospice concept "stands as a protest against the shortcomings of modern high technology medicine," and he adds, "We are witnessing an attempt to re-emphasize that doctors, nurses and para-medicals are in business 'to cure sometime, to relieve often, to comfort always.' "

Let me quote you a section of a presentation Dr. Twycross gave at a 1979 Anglo-American Conference on Care of the Dying:

"In terminal illness, the primary aim is no longer to preserve life, but to make the life that remains as comfortable and as meaningful as possible. Thus, what may be appropriate treatment in an acutely ill patient may be inappropriate in the dying.

"Cardiac resuscitation, artificial respiration, intravenous infusions, nasogastric tubes, antibiotics—all are primarily supportive measures for use in acute illnesses to assist a patient through the initial period toward recovery of health. To use such measures in the terminally ill, with no expectancy of a return to health, is generally inappropriate and is—therefore—bad medicine by definition.

"It is, however, not a question of 'to treat or not to treat?' but of what is appropriate treatment from a biological point of view in the light of the patient's personal and social circumstances."

In the past ten years, the hospice approach to care of the terminally ill has developed in various parts of North America. Dr. Sylvia Lack, medical director of the Connecticut Hospice in Hew Haven, put it succinctly in a recent paper: "We are not involved in the business of killing people. We are in the business of improving the quality of remaining life, which involves making the distinction between appropriate and inappropriate treatment for patients."

The New Haven facility has a home-care program and a forty-bed inpatient hospital patterned on the British model. Other groups—some two hundred at last count—in the United States and Canada are putting the same principles into operation using the same or different methods.

For example, the Palliative Care Service of the Royal Victoria Hospital in Montreal has a limited number of beds within a general hospital. The unit concentrates on deliverying hospice care in conjunction with a home-care program.

Saint Luke's Hospital in New York City has a hospice interdisciplinary team made up of doctors, nurses, social workers, and chaplains who work together visiting terminal patients within the hospital. Together, this group works for the improvement of symptom control, to provide family and home care, to give twenty-four-hour coverage, and to handle all the other aspects of the hospice approach.

Dr. Cecily Saunders points out that control of physical pain is not the whole picture in hospice care.

Often the symptoms of illness are also an embarrassment and a source of mental distress to the patient, leading to such reactions as shame, anxiety, depression, and bitterness.

Dr. Saunders found that the staff could help by attending to such obvious problems as nausea, vomiting, shortness of breath, oral pain, diarrhea, and constipation. The patient may become totally weary of the whole process, feeling depressed and guilty—which in turn leads to a kind of self-hostility. These feelings may be projected outward, appearing as resentment of those who care for the person.

For this reason Dr. Saunders found it important to give attention to the family. One of the best ways was to recruit them as part of the caring team and give them the opportunity to voice their feelings, whether guilt, weariness, or impatience. In this way the final bereavement was eased.

Our forefathers knew more about their own spiritual needs than many a college-educated high-intellect graduate of today. They knew that man is by nature a creature of ritual, made insecure by rapid change, fearful of the unknown, yet creative enough to people it with imaginary terrors more awful than reality.

Ritual serves to soothe the insecurity of change; rites of passage give a firmer anchor to the identity; practice of the known eases acceptance of the unknown. Our planet is littered with memorials to this view, mausoleums not for the dead but as an ever-present comfort to the living.

The old-fashioned undertaker—hardy businessman though he was—knew that ritualized grief eased the tension of bereavement by giving a sense of things accomplished, of work done. Hence his insistence, scorned of late, on the proprieties—wreaths, cards, lying in state, viewing, and the assembly of family and friends in the somber funeral ritual.

The undertaker made his money from it. But the bereaved got what they paid for—a funeral that left no doubt in anyone's mind that the deceased had been permanently removed from the community with a dignity befitting the passing of a loved one.

Advances in psychology and counseling techniques have given us less ponderous means of easing the processes of social change, but we should be wary of simply dispensing with ritual without adequate provision for channeling the forces that power the psyche.

During my public debate with Dr. Saunders, a speaker from the floor queried the "enormous expense" of the hospice system. It was the first time in a two-hour long, fairly abrasive discussion that the doctor almost lost her cool.

Speaking slowly and clearly, as if keeping a tight rein on her emotions but anxious that there should be no misunderstanding of the depth of her feeling on the subject, she made it clear that a society that could not afford to care for the dying placed little value on human life.

I subscribe to that view, not because I am moving into the late summer of my life and have had a hint of the chill winds of autumn. I do so because I have come to realize that a life without values, of which humane consideration for others must surely be a basic, is no life at all.

What separates man from beast are not his gadgets and his gimmicks, but a disciplined way of viewing life and the ability to know what is worthwhile in human terms and what is mere biological existence.

When my time comes, I ask only that I will know the difference and still have the option of terminating before one shades into the other.

Four

Throughout history, the concept of medical euthanasia—terminating a life as an extension of the medical treatment of a dying patient—has had little public acceptance. For that reason, we can well ask if it is possible for society—legislators, religious leaders, the man on the street—to reach a consensus on the acceptable practice of euthanasia.

At present, it seems unlikely. But recently other weighty medicolegal problems have weathered extensive and heated discussions and suffered a sea change after sound judgment prevailed.

I speak of euthanasia as derived from its original Greek context, meaning an easy or painless death. In recent years, two types of euthanasia have been mentioned in professional discussions of termination of life. One is called active, or direct (in which life is ended by direct intervention, such as giving a patient a lethal dose of a drug). The other is referred to as passive, or indirect (with death resulting from withdrawal of life-support systems or life-sustaining medications).

Later we will consider both types of euthanasia more specifically. Before we do, however, I would like to show how times, and medical thinking, do change.

Even the revered Hippocratic oath, for instance, has undergone some alteration. Although for generations the oath has been a traditional aspect of medical school graduation ceremonies, some schools have abandoned it altogether; others have substituted the Declaration of Geneva—adopted in 1914 by the World Medical Association; still others have made word changes.

Recently, the American College of Physicians surveyed schools on the North American continent to get an idea of current attitudes. In Canada, where only a few schools use the Hippocratic oath (see Appendix), a dean replied, "There is a danger that a college administering such an oath would tend to absolve itself of responsibility for the student and graduate's future ethical and moral conduct on the basis that it had administered the oath."

The original Oath of Hippocrates had a section relating to both euthanasia and abortion, which many of the younger generation of medical students find to be out of step with the 1980s: "I will give no deadly medicine to anyone if asked, nor suggest any such counsel; furthermore, I will not give to a woman an instrument to produce abortion."

The abortion issue came to the fore at the University of Pittsburgh in 1971 when graduating medical students switched from the Hippocratic oath to the Declaration of Geneva. First, however, they deleted the words "from the time of conception" from the clause beginning "I will maintain the utmost respect for human life."

Perhaps there will never be complete consensus on the rights and wrongs of abortion. The arguments, pro and con, would fill volumes, and there seems no end in sight to the controversy.

In consideration of the ethics of abortion, the American Medical Association (AMA) has offered guidance to its membership by indicating that abortion is a "medical procedure." In 1974, the AMA's House of Delegates supported "the right of the American people to be free from coercion in determining when they will submit to the performance of elective medical procedures such as sterilization and abortion."

This policy statement went further, and I think rightfully so, by adding that no physician or hospital staff member "shall be required to perform an act violative of good medical judgement or personally held moral principles."

For my part, a Calvinistic upbringing does not allow me to accept the idea of "free" abortion, in which the fetus is aborted simply because it is not convenient for a woman to have a baby.

On the other hand, it is clear to me that there are times when a doctor might conclude that a woman's life can be saved, or the *quality* of her life preserved, if she has an abortion. Or that by terminating a pregnancy—of a mongoloid fetus, for example—a child doomed to a life without quality would not, indeed, be born.

Another example of a heated debate on a medicolegal issue stemmed from my early work in heart transplantation. A worldwide commentary and controversy was triggered in an effort to determine the ultimate question: When is a person dead?

The issue was first broached in modern form in 1957 when, at the International Congress of Anesthesiologists in Rome, Pope Pius XII was asked, "When does death occur?"

The pope's reply was that "human life continues for as long as its vital functions, distinguished from the simple life of the organs, manifest themselves spontaneously without the help of artificial processes." He added that the task of determining the "exact instant of death" was that of the physician.

He did not clarify whether he meant that the medical profession had the responsibility of deciding precisely which bodily functions were essential to continued life, or whether he was saying simply that it was up to the doctor to determine when those functions had ceased in a particular patient.

In any event, Pope Pius XII seemed to have placed a special responsibility on the physician's shoulders, for he pointed out that doctors are not bound to use extraordinary measures to prolong life when it is impossible to consult the patient. He also noted that life-shortening drugs could be used to relieve unbearable pain, "provided no other means exist."

Debate continues on another point he raised: If attempts at resuscitation and prolongation of life work an undue hardship on the patient's family, "they can rightly insist that the doctor interrupt his efforts."

Although these pronouncements upheld, in effect, the patient's right to die, they brought us no nearer to the means of determining when death actually occurs.

One of the earliest systematic examinations of the matter was carried out just after the first heart transplants by a committee of Harvard University scholars. Formed early in 1968, the Ad Hoc Committee to Examine the Definition of Brain Death included physicians, theologians, lawyers, and philosophers. The need to establish such a definition related to criticism suggesting that heart transplant surgeons might remove a vital donor organ from a patient not yet dead.

Among the key recommendations made by the committee was one that previous definitions of death had either applied or hinted at: A patient is dead when the brain is dead, or when the patient has gone into irreversible coma.

Specifically, four grounds for the definition of death were recommended as follows:

1. *Unreceptivity and lack of responsiveness.* There is a total unawareness to externally applied stimuli and inner need, and complete unresponsiveness—irreversible coma. Even the most painful stimuli evoke no vocal or other response, not even a groan, withdrawal of a limb, or quickening of respiration.

2. *No movement or breathing.* Observation by physicians, covering a period of at least one hour, is adequate to satisfy the criteria of no spontaneous muscular movements, no spontaneous respiration, and no response to stimuli such as pain, touch, sound, or light.

3. *No reflexes.* Irreversible coma with abolition of central nervous system activity is evidenced in part by the

absence of elicitable reflexes. The pupil will be fixed and dilated and will not respond to a direct source of bright light.

4. *Flat encephalogram.* Of great confirmatory value is the flat or isoelectric EEG. We must assume that the electrodes have been properly applied, that the apparatus is functioning normally, and that the staff in charge is competent.

In applying these guidelines to clinical practice—for instance, when the decision has to be made as to whether or not to remove life-support systems from a patient—the Harvard scholars recommended that when the brain is obviously dead, using the recommended criteria, two physicians (one a neurologist or a neurosurgeon) might agree to inform the patient's family that the respirator should be turned off.

"It is pointless and needlessly cruel to ask the family to make this decision," the committee stated.

Only at this stage, the committee urged, should physicians involved in organ transplantation enter the picture—if they are to be involved at all. In that case, artificial respiration may be continued, almost indefinitely, to preserve the viability of organs required for transplantation.

The Harvard committee recommendations have probably had the most far-reaching effect of any set of guidelines and have been reflected to some degree or another in virtually all the codes of practice since adopted or proposed.

Of course, these recommendations reflected the widespread medical-scientific opinion of the time.

Some two months before publication of the committee's findings, a meeting of thirteen cardiac surgeons in Cape Town agreed that brain death should be the accepted criterion for death.

The cardiac surgeons pointed out that there should be no sign of cerebral activity, but they did not specify the length of time during which the patient should be kept under observation for that activity.

In most of the heart transplants that were carried out in the first few months after the procedure was introduced, there had been a flat EEG in the donor for more than two hours. In other words, those of us doing heart transplants had already arrived at a working definition of death based on the presence or absence of cerebral activity.

Even earlier, a month before the Cape Town meeting, the Council of the Organization of Medical Science—which met in Geneva—came up with guidelines very much like those worked out by the Harvard group.

The criteria for the cessation of cerebral function, or death, set forth by the council were as follows:

1. Loss of all response to the environment.

2. Complete loss of reflexes and muscle tone.

3. Absence of spontaneous respiration.

4. Massive drop in arterial blood pressure when not artificially maintained.

5. Even with artificial stimulation of the brain, an absolutely linear electroencephalographic tracing recorded under the best technical conditions.

Two months later, or at about the time that the Harvard recommendations appeared in print, the World Medical Assembly—meeting in Sydney—adopted a statement on death that seemed to sidestep the problem of precise definition.

The Sydney Declaration read:

"The determination of the time of death in most countries is the legal responsibility of the physician and should remain so. A complication is that death is a gradual process at the cellular level with tissues varying in their ability to withstand deprivation of oxygen. But clinical interest lies not in the state of preservation of isolated cells, but in the fate of the person. Here the point of death of the different cells and organs is not as important as the certainty that the process has become irreversible by whatever techniques of resuscitation that may be employed.

"This determination may be based on clinical judgement, supplemented if necessary by a number of diagnostic aids, of which the electroencephalograph is currently the most helpful. However, no single technological criterion is entirely satisfactory in the present state of medicine, nor can one technological procedure be substituted for the overall judgement of the physician. If transplantation is involved, the decision that death exists should be made by two or more physicians, and the physician determining the moment of death should in no way be immediately concerned with the performance of transplantation."

Certainly, in the eyes of many, this declaration had the advantage over some of its predecessors of not tying determination of death to any single test or procedure. Instead, it seems to say that the moment of death shall be determined by the best available means at a given time and place.

At the time, the president of the assembly, Sir Leonard Mallen, said, "With scientific advances and new methods of resuscitation always coming up, it would be silly of us to give a definition which could be outmoded within half an hour."

Indeed, it quickly became apparent that too rigid a definition of death might be as troublesome as older concepts appear to be in the age of seemingly miraculous resuscitative technology and organ transplantation. It was early pointed out, for example, that a flat electroencephalogram is not really a prerequisite for judging a patient's death.

There is the further problem that not all hospitals where people die will necessarily have an electroencephalograph. Often when such a machine is available, there is no technical expertise to determine that the apparently flat EEG really indicates cerebral death.

Alternative investigative laboratory procedures to the use of the electroencephalograph have been proposed. These include cerebral angiography and measures of cerebral circulation and/or metabolism. The usual rationale for these added measures is that they may provide additional protection against declaration of death merely on the evidence of a flat EEG.

In my view, the reason for error in the diagnosis of brain death is usually obvious. Most often, there has been a confusion between brain death as such and irreversible brain damage leading to the vegetative state.

Patients in the vegetative state are not dependent on a ventilator, in spite of permanent and irreversible damage to the cerebral cortex and the inability ever to function again as human beings. Such persons may live for months or even years without major life-support systems.

How long support should be continued for these unfortunates—the truly vegetative person as opposed to the brain dead—is another matter. It should not further confuse the already confused question of brain death.

Failure to diagnose brain death has occasionally been made on the basis of continued spinal reflexes. However, these reflexes may continue after brain death—particularly in patients who have received depressant drugs or where the body temperature has fallen to subnormal levels before death.

This kind of situation commonly arises in cases where the patient has been admitted to the emergency room after being found unconscious and no medical history is available. It is in these circumstances that various specialist opinions and highly technical laboratory procedures come into play—not so much to determine whether or not the patient is dead, or brain dead, but to diagnose the cause of the difficulty and try to remedy it.

Even in this situation, the cause of the unresponsiveness may be obvious. The patient's head may be crushed, or it may become clear within perhaps half an hour that the person has had a prolonged period of heart stoppage or maybe a stroke. Sometimes the combination of an underlying disease and a recent stroke or heart attack will put the matter beyond hope.

In such cases, the individual physician may move with a calculated slowness in starting up resuscitation procedures. For if he manages to resuscitate the patient, there may be difficulty in stopping the resuscitative measures.

In 1976, possibly reflecting the dilemmas posed for the physician in these circumstances, two Boston hospitals made public their policies in handling the hopelessly ill.

The Massachusetts General Hospital policy—known as Optimum Care for Hopelessly Ill Patients—was the work of the hospital's Critical Care Committee. In addition to a number of physicians, nurses, a psychiatrist, an attorney, and a Jesuit priest, this group included a woman who had recovered from cancer.

Under this policy, patients were classified on admission into categories, based on the likelihood of their survival. The strenuousness of resuscitative care and/or therapeutic effort was graduated accordingly.

The groups were listed as follows:

1. Maximal therapeutic effort without reservation.

2. The same, but "with daily evaluation because the probability of survival is questionable."

3. Selective limitation of therapeutic measures. In such instances, there might be orders not to resuscitate, or to withhold antibiotics in an apparently terminal pneumonia.

4. All therapy can be discontinued. This category includes patients with brain death as well as those who have no chance of regaining "cognitive and sapient life," i.e., those facing a vegetative existence.

In theory, at least, the responsible physician has the basic authority over the patient's treatment, extending to the right to reject the advice of the hospital committee. However, the director of the hospital's intensive care unit is empowered to take the matter either to his chief of service or to the Critical Care Committee itself if it seems warranted.

This poses the possibility of tangled lines of responsibility between primary physician and hospital staff—one of the main criticisms of the Massachusetts General Hospital's approach. On the face of it, there seems little room—or at least no specific role—for the patient's family in what are clearly life and death decisions.

The committee rules do state that "no definite act of commission"—such as shutting down a respirator—may be carried out before the family has agreed. The guidelines seem to have been written on the assumption that most patients who are sufficiently ill for the consideration of cessation of treatment will be comatose at the time the question comes up.

The primary physician and hospital staff, it would appear, are given the major responsibility for setting the approach to the patient. However, the burden of permission for the acts that implement that approach may devolve on the family.

On the other hand, a second Boston hospital, Beth Israel, has announced a policy that appears to emphasize the patient's right to decide what should be done about his own care. The committee dealing with the care of the hopelessly ill in this case would seem to limit its activity to advising the primary physician on whether the death of his patient is so imminent or foregone that resuscitation would serve no useful purpose.

However, once such a decision has been made

on physiological grounds, the responsibility for actually issuing orders to implement the policy would shift to the patient and/or family. The important point is that where there is no such consent, the policy, or order not to resuscitate, could not be carried out.

Whatever an institution's policy toward the hopelessly ill, it is clear that it will reflect the attitude of the institution toward the diagnosis of death. It is also clear that something approaching brain death, however determined, is the central theme in most recent criteria for the determination of death.

A more recent attempt by an important medical body to lay down guidelines for determining death came from the Conference of Medical Royal Colleges and their Faculties, in the United Kingdom. This set of rules, published in 1976, was prepared in consultation with the Royal College of Physicians, the Faculty of Anaesthetists, and the Royal College of Surgeons.

The diagnostic criteria set out "are accepted as being sufficient to distinguish between those patients who retain the functional capacity to have a chance of even partial recovery from those in whom no such possibility exists."

Briefly, the criteria are as follows:

1. The patient is deeply comatose. Here, possible effects of depressant drugs, hypothermia (abnormally low body temperature), and the like can be ruled out.

2. The patient is being maintained on a ventilator because spontaneous respiration had previously become inadequate or had ceased altogether. Here again, the effects of various drugs such as relaxants, hypnotics, and narcotics can be ruled out.

3. There should be no doubt that the patient's condition is due to irremediable structural brain damage. The diagnosis of a disorder that can lead to brain death should be fully established.

The Conference's report explained, "It may be obvious within hours of a primary intracranial event such as severe head injury, spontaneous intracranial hemorrhage, or after neurosurgery that the condition is irremediable. But when a patient has suffered primarily from cardiac arrest, hypoxia, or severe circulatory insufficiency with an indefinite period of cerebral anoxia or is suspected of having cerebral air or fat embolism, then it may take much longer to establish the diagnosis and to be confident of the prognosis. In some patients the primary condition may be a matter of doubt and a confident diagnosis may be reached only by continuous clinical observation and investigation."

The recommendations of the Medical Royal Colleges and Faculties are notable in several respects. For one thing, they do not specify the particular tests to be done or the interval at which they should be done.

The test or evaluation interval should depend on "the primary condition and the clinical course of the disease." In certain conditions, it would even be unnecessary to repeat tests, "since a prognosis of imminent death can be accepted as being obvious." In other cases, the outcome may be less obvious, and the interval between tests might be as much as twenty-four hours.

Another point worth noting is that, unlike the

Harvard committee guidelines, the Medical Royal Colleges criteria do not explicitly endorse use of the electroencephalograph. "It is now widely accepted that electroencephalography is not necessary for diagnosing brain death," they explained.

"Electroencephalography has its principal value at earlier stages in the care of patients when the original diagnosis is in doubt. When an EEG is called for, then the strict criteria recommended by the Federation of EEG Societies must be followed. Other investigations such as cerebral angiography or cerebral blood flow measurements are not required for diagnosing brain death."

The Colleges' recommendations make no reference to organ transplantation. This omission, it has been pointed out, underscores the fact that brain death is common whereas the issue of organ donation arises only infrequently.

In 1978 the Department of Health in Britain sent copies of the Colleges' recommendations to every doctor in the country. With each copy went a covering letter to the effect that lack of criticism since publication of the criteria suggested that they had already been widely accepted within the medical profession.

The letter also emphasized that the diagnosis of brain death must be reached entirely independently of transplant considerations, and "it must remain absolutely clear that this is so."

Once the diagnosis of death has been made, however, the actual moment at which a respirator can be switched off may be influenced by the need to keep organs in the best possible condition for transplantation.

As the law now stands in Britain, a person is dead when a doctor declares him so. There are no hard-and-fast rules to tell the doctor how he may arrive at this decision.

In the United States, in spite of efforts on the part of state legislators to set forth legal criteria for determining death, as well as numerous court decisions interpreting such laws (or more commonly the absence thereof), the situation is not greatly different.

The attempts made to codify and update the old common-law attitudes toward death in general closely paralleled efforts made by the medical profession to establish criteria for determining death. But, although guidelines laid down by the medical profession usually took pains to eschew any link between a determination of brain death and possible organ transplantation, many—perhaps most—of the laws enacted by the individual states were expressly designed to facilitate transplantation.

The first, and by all accounts the model, state statute laying down rules for diagnosing death was enacted by Kansas in 1970. This law establishes two alternative "definitions of death," as follows:

"A person will be considered medically and legally dead if, in the opinion of a physician based on ordinary medical standards of medical practice, there is the absence of spontaneous respiratory and cardiac function and, because of the disease or condition which caused directly or indirectly these functions to cease, or because of the passage of time since these functions ceased, attempts at resuscitation are considered hopeless; and in this event death will have occurred at the time these functions ceased; or

"A person will be considered medically and legally dead if, in the opinion of a physician based on ordinary standards of medical practice, there is absence of spontaneous brain function; and if based on ordinary standards of medical practice, during reasonable attempts to either maintain or restore spontaneous circulatory or respiratory function in the absence of aforesaid brain function, it appears that further attempts at resuscitation or supportive maintenance will not succeed, death will have occurred at the time when these conditions coincide. Death is to be pronounced before artificial means of supporting respiratory and circulatory function are terminated and before any vital organ is removed for purpose of transplantation."

In Kansas, these alternative definitions of death are to be utilized for all purposes—including the trials of civil and criminal cases.

By the beginning of 1980, some twenty-five states had adopted some form of legislation concerning brain death. The American Medical Association has come up with a model law (see Appendix) and is encouraging physicians to promote its passage by state legislatures.

Interestingly, most of the objection to such legislation seems to have come from the legal profession. One British attorney commented, "By all means let us have guidelines. They are essential. But let them be set down by the medical profession."

Another objection is that the laws patterned after the Kansas statute seem to have been written with transplantation specifically in mind, as opposed to updating the criteria for death. This appears to have been the case with the original Kansas law, as the

University of Kansas Medical Center was very interested in transplants at the time and staff members were advocating a change in the law.

Another related objection centers on the proviso that death be pronounced before artificial respiration and circulation are discontinued, just as the original Harvard recommendations specified. According to this objection, the main point is not that this shouldn't be done, but that it shouldn't be enshrined in law.

The law, it is reasoned, may not be the proper place for spelling out in technical detail the steps a physician should take in declaring a patient dead.

As for turning off the respirator and ventilatory support only after death has been pronounced, this is done and has been done by physicians on an individual basis ever since advanced life-support systems became available. At times it was done to facilitate transplantation, but in most instances, I would stress, it has nothing to do with transplantation.

But whether it has or not, courts in the United States have fairly consistently recognized and upheld brain death as the major criterion in the determination of the moment of death. In most cases, it is well to emphasize, it has been brain death as determined by the physician using medically acceptable norms—as opposed to any particular technique such as a flat encephalogram.

Most surprisingly, one of the earliest court cases to examine the concept of brain death involved transplantation—and a heart transplant at that.

Early in 1968, surgeons at the Medical College

of Virginia, led by the eminent cardiac surgeon Dr. David M. Hume, had in their hospital an ideal candidate for heart transplantation. As it happened, shortly after the cardiac patient was admitted, a forty-year-old laborer suffered massive brain damage in an accident.

Except for an occasional artifact caused by the electronic circuit itself, the accident victim's electroencephalogram was flat. The patient was continued on a respirator, however, and his body temperature, pulse, and blood pressure all remained normal for a man in his condition.

Toward midafternoon, the laborer was taken to the operating theater and prepared for removal of his heart and kidneys. Oxygen was given to ensure the continued viability of these organs. The court record shows that body temperature, blood pressure, and respiration continued normal for the circumstances.

At 3:30 P.M., the respirator was shut off. Five minutes later the man was pronounced dead, and the respirator was restarted to preserve the heart and kidneys. The heart was removed and transplanted into the cardiac patient.

The record shows that no attempt was made to get permission from any of the accident victim's relatives for any of the procedures, in spite of the fact that his wallet contained the address and phone number of a brother who worked some fifteen blocks from the hospital.

Since, as the trial judge later pointed out, Virginia law then defined death as the total cessation of all bodily functions, the laborer's brother brought suit against the surgical team for wrongfully ending a life.

The suit, in effect, alleged that the accident victim had been alive when the heart was removed and that in doing so the surgeons had killed him.

During the trial the physicians maintained that, using the criteria of brain death, the heart donor had actually been dead for several hours before the heart was removed. The jury concurred that a man whose brain was dead was indeed dead.

The judge in this case had instructed the jury that they might use either the classical definition of death or the newer one. But at the same time he noted that the jury would need to decide whether the life-support machines were maintaining the classic signs of life.

Ironically, in Massachusetts itself—where the Harvard committee came up with one of the earliest formulations of the brain death principle—the courts recognized it only recently. The case involved was not concerned with transplantation, but it is worth recounting for its own interest.

The issue came up in the murder trial of an eighteen-year-old youth who had attacked a thirty-four-year-old man from behind. He had struck the man over the head with a baseball bat and left him lying there in the street. In court, he said he did not know the man and had done it "just for kicks."

The assault victim had been rushed to the hospital. His skull had been smashed in, and a large part of it had to be removed to relieve pressure on the brain. He was placed on a respirator.

Since complete recovery seemed unlikely, tests for brain function were carried out. He showed no blood pressure, and heartbeat and pulse were undetectable. The respirator was disconnected for two minutes, and he did not breathe.

Two days later, the tests were repeated. Again the EEG was flat; there were no reflexes, and no responses could be detected. When the respirator was once more turned off momentarily, the man again did not breathe spontaneously.

After consultation with the victim's family, the respirator was disconnected three days later.

The assailant's attorney, relying on the traditional definition of death, contended that the action of the victim's physicians and family had interfered with normal life processes and had deprived his client of a possible defense. The attorney appeared to be saying, in effect, that there was no telling how long the man might have lived had the respirator not been disconnected.

At the trial, various expert witnesses explained that the medical community generally accepted the criterion of brain death as the key to determining the actual point of demise. The attending physician said that he had felt that the patient had died some five days before the respirator was disconnected. He also testified that the disconnection of the respirator for the last time was "in accordance with good medical practice." The local medical examiner testified that in his opinion the man had died three days before the respirator was disconnected.

The judge specifically charged the jury in the case to apply the test of brain death. He defined the concept as occurring when, in the opinion of a licensed physician using ordinary and accepted standards of medical practice, total and irreversible cessation of brain function has taken place, and further attempts at resuscitation would be unsuccessful in restarting those functions.

It is immediately apparent that the judge did not include any of the technical criteria that might be used by the physician in making a judgment. To this extent, he was applying one of the alternatives laid down earlier by the Kansas statute.

Two questions were to be decided by the jury: (1) Was the brain death concept satisfied by the evidence in the case? and (2) Did the victim die before or after the life-support mechanism was disconnected for the last time?

The jury affirmed the first question and concluded that death had actually occurred before the respirator was disconnected.

Clearly, it now appears that the medical profession and such laws on the matter as have been enacted in the Western world, as well as in the courts of law, all recognize and accept the concept of brain death.

More importantly, it also appears that the diagnosis of brain death need not be arrived at by any specific means or tests, but may simply be determined by the attending physician acting according to accepted medical norms.

We have come a long way since Pope Pius XII set forth his opinion on determination of death. And the courts of law are only now beginning to establish legal precedence.

Perhaps, at some time in the future, the same road will be followed in establishing guidelines (both medical and legal) for the acceptable practice of active or passive termination of life—euthanasia.

48

——Five——

Medical science knows much more about death than about life. Death can be accurately diagnosed, although when it is present, the doctor can do little more than console the family to the best of his ability.

On the other hand, even though life does not lend itself to an easy definition, it is the doctor's duty to give his patient a good life. After all, the goal of medicine is to improve the quality of life or arrest the deterioration in quality where this has been set in motion by a disease process.

As long as the disease responds to medical or surgical treatment, there is no problem. The moral dilemma arises when, in spite of all treatment, the quality of life falls and there is an increase in physical suffering.

Should the doctor now attempt, with all the means at his disposal, to prolong the existence of the patient? I use the term *existence* because it is debatable whether the patient is still truly alive.

Or, from that point onward, should the doctor concentrate on improving the quality of dying, even if this may hasten the death of the patient?

During the terminal illness of President Tito of Yugoslavia, the whole world was made aware of the incongruity of a human body existing without truly "living." Here was a man who lived a good life—a great life by the standards of mankind—whose death was abated by life supports and by the ministrations of a team of doctors.

Over a period of many weeks after his left leg was amputated, the news media duly reported Mr. Tito's deterioration. It was almost a compendium of serious ailments—any one of which could bring about the end of life. One bulletin issued by his physicians said that the President was in a coma most of the time, with wildly fluctuating body temperatures. He suffered from "heavy stomach bleeding, heart weakness, cardiac rhythm disturbances, kidney failure, pneumonia and diabetes."

The Houston Post, in an editorial, rightfully called the situation a "doctors' dilemma." The editorial said, in part:

"After his surgery [President Tito] seemed sufficiently on the road to recovery to warrant first one, then another, life-saving emergency measure. To have denied them would have been unethical and not in keeping with modern medical practice. At the time, he and his doctors were averse to the idea of prolonging his life artificially should he become terminally ill. But gradually, as one machine after another replaced a function of his body, Tito began to sink. He is now in a coma. It is fairly sure that he is being kept alive only by the massive system of life-support equipment. Nothing now can reverse the progress of his illness or restore him to consciousness, much less to a precarious health.

"It is probable that his protracted illness has allowed time in Belgrade for political forces to resolve their differences and plan an orderly transition. But the physicians in charge face a question: Do they continue to keep alive a man who can no longer live in any real sense of the word? If not, who will make the decision to withdraw the supports?"

I have said earlier that death does not concern me, but dying does. This leads me to define my view of euthanasia as not so much a good death as a comfortable dying. To me it certainly does not mean mercy killing. Yet I hold strongly that medicine cannot shirk its responsibilities during this period of the patient's existence.

There are those who believe that no one has the right to hasten a patient's death, that man should not play God—ever.

But a physician, as a scientist, must live in a world of reality. The dogmatic attitude toward euthanasia reminds me of the condition of pregnancy—an all or nothing state. In short, you cannot be slightly pregnant.

A dogmatic approach sees only one point, either black or white, and loses out on all the shades of gray in between.

In considering the application of current thought toward the so-called "good death," a doctor is inclined to muse on the years spent in hospital wards, as a physician in training, as a struggling surgeon, as a teacher making the rounds—surrounded always by a sea of patients ranging from the convalescent to the terminally ill.

There is joy in dealing with those who will recover, but your heart goes out to the child you know will not live the night; your eyes mist when you see a weeping husband at the end of visiting hours saying good-bye to his cancer-ridden wife, perhaps for the last time.

In such circumstances, it is hard to believe that any comforting action taken by a physician—even to the extent that it hastens death—is wrong. And you are painfully aware that, in spite of opinions expressed by members of the medical profession, most doctors know deep in their hearts that euthanasia is the right form of treatment for some terminally ill patients.

Indeed, even though many doctors will not admit it, passive euthanasia is accepted medical practice—a common occurrence in wards where patients live out their final hours.

There lies the patient with terminal cancer, the body riddled with secondary spread; deeply sedated, barely alive. Suddenly, the patient develops a cardiac arrest. If the doctor does not start cardiac massage immediately and shock the heart back to a beating state, is he withholding treatment?

It is such a thin line. Is it wrong to allow death and peace to come? Or is it unethical to intervene at this point to allow the patient to see another day of suffering?

In another ward, a family stands around the bed of a patient who is being kept alive by a respirator. The heart monitor machine confirms, in its eerie audible way, that the heart is still beating. But the doctor knows that life has really ended—there is no recognition, no awareness, nor will there ever be.

After a final assessment of the situation and a discussion with the relatives, the medical team decides not to continue a life that no longer has meaning. A switch is clicked, a dial turned. Life support stops, and in a matter of minutes the pulse on the heart monitor flattens and the staccato bleep becomes a monotone hum.

Was the doctors' decision to flick the switch a form of killing or was it good medical treatment—an act of mercy? That scene by the bedside is no different from one that has been played out on occasion in the operating rooms of many hospitals. Every heart surgeon who has practiced for any length of time has gone through the following nightmare:

The patient is on the operating table, the chest cavity open and the diseased heart exposed. Surrounding the patient is machinery—miracles of modern technology: a respirator breathing life-sustaining oxygen into the lungs, a monitor translating bodily functions into visual patterns on the view screens, and the heart-lung machine, the technological advance that made open-heart surgery possible.

At some point during the surgical procedure, this machine will be connected to the circulation of the patient in preparation for taking over the function of the heart and lungs, thus allowing the surgeon to open any chamber of the heart and expose its interior.

When the connections are complete, the surgeon gives the command, "pump on." The heart-lung technician throws a switch, and slowly the heart empties as the impure blood returning from the body is diverted through the machine. Oxygen is then bubbled through the blue blood, driving off the impurities and turning it red again as the oxygen is replenished. From this point, the blood is pumped back through the patient's own circulation.

"Stop the respirator," is the surgeon's next command. The anesthesiologist operates a switch, and the bellows of the mechanical respirator deflate. The patient's lungs come to rest.

At this stage, both circulation and respiration are totally taken over by the machine, but the heart is still beating.

"Cool the patient, clamp on the aorta, start running the cardioplegic solution [heart paralyzing fluid]." The heartbeat falters, stops. The heart muscle becomes soft and relaxed.

The heart is not beating, the lungs are not breathing, but the patient is alive—held in this state by the heart-lung machine supplying oxygenated blood to the patient's brain.

The operation is difficult. Major defects, unsuspected even after exhaustive preoperative testing, come to light when the heart is opened. In such surgery the risks are always high—and the odds sometimes win.

In my early years as a young surgeon I worked with men who, when faced with such odds, would virtually rewrite the textbook in terms of brilliant surgery performed on the operating table.

But when all has been done that can be done, there remains the unspoken bottom-line question: Will the repaired heart react under the strain of full circulation when unsupported by the heart machine?

"Aortic clamp off."

"Rewarm the patient."

Warm oxygenated blood returns to the cold oxygen-deprived heart muscles. The heart pinks up and becomes tense, then the muscle fibers each start to contract in an uncoordinated rhythm.

"Defibrillator."

The electrodes are handed to the surgeon, who applies them to the surface of the heart.

"Shock."

The patient's body jerks briefly. The heart muscle fibers stop for a second and then, miraculously, begin coordinated contraction.

"Partial bypass."

The heart-lung technician allows some of the venous blood to flow back into the heart and reduces the circulatory support from the machine. The chambers of the heart fill up. The beat, though not as vigorous as before, continues.

"Start the ventilator."

The anesthesiologist turns a switch, and the bellows of the mechanical respirator begin pumping oxygen back into the patient's lungs.

"Stop the heart-lung machine."

The patient is on his own. There is no circulatory support.

The heart swells, begins to struggle. The beat slows. It is clear it cannot handle the full circulatory load. The heart-lung machine is switched on again to support circulation, and drugs are given to tone up the heart muscle. Soon a vigorous contraction returns.

Again the support of the heart-lung machine is reduced and eventually stopped. The heart falters and fails again. The procedure is repeated. An hour passes, and other complicating factors make their appearance, not the least being the accumulative damage caused to the delicate blood cells as they pass through the heart pump. No matter how sophisticatedly fashioned, no machine can fully mimic the action of the human heart.

Less traumatic partial mechanical support is instituted without success. Owing to the fact that throughout the long struggle sufficient oxygen has been supplied to the brain, the patient is still alive, but the medical team has exhausted all available means at its disposal to return the patient to a life of acceptable quality.

Finally, for the last time, the heart-lung machine is switched off. The heart fails and stops beating. The oxygen level in the brain drops; brain activity ceases. The patient is dead.

It can be argued that the surgeon's command to stop the heart-lung machine killed the patient. Alternatively, it could be said that the surgeon gave the patient, who could no longer have a good life, a good death.

This emotionally draining experience led me to think long and hard about the possibilities of some kind of heart assist that would avoid the problems of the mechanical pump. The result was the development, at Groote Schuur, of the twin-heart, or piggyback, technique of transplant in which a donor heart is used to assist the failing heart rather than to replace it.

It seemed logical to assume that a second heart, helping the load carried by a malfunctioning organ, would return a patient to a good quality life. Further, the rest given to a patient's heart after the trauma of surgery would often allow it to return to full function. If later tests showed this to be the case, then the second heart could be removed and the patient would be able to live as good a life as would have been possible if his own heart had been able to take over immediately.

I was very excited about this concept. Few people realize the total loneliness of the surgeon when a patient, as the expression goes, "dies on the table." There is a feeling of complete inadequacy as the doctor pulls off his gloves and mask and walks out to the waiting room to explain to the relatives what happened.

There was one major problem attached to putting the twin-heart concept into practice—the nonavailability of donor hearts on an instant-call basis. In spite of full preoperative investigations, it is very difficult to predict which patients will run into trouble after correction of a heart lesion; therefore, the need for a donor heart under these circumstances is generally an emergency. The donor must be available immediately and, even in the largest of hospitals, this is seldom possible.

Perhaps a digression is in order here to explain why the first heart transplant was carried out in South Africa and not by a team in other parts of the world such as the United States.

It was not because we were better prepared than surgeons elsewhere but because it was generally assumed that the first human heart transplant could only be performed in an emergency situation and in the circumstances I have described. In December 1967, we decided to do it as a scheduled cold case in a patient dying from irreversible destruction of the heart muscle—a terminal state not responsive to medical treatment—as soon as a donor became available.

Since that time, the availability of donors has been a major stumbling block in heart transplant programs around the world. Because of this fact, when the concept of the piggyback transplant became an established technique, we decided to explore the possibility of using the heart of another primate—such as a baboon or a chimpanzee. Suitable animals were readily available in South Africa and could be kept near the hospital.

Although we realized that rejection of the heart would be a major problem, our laboratory tests indicated that—with the drugs available—it might be possible to protect the donor animal heart against the immunological onslaught of the patient's body for a few days. In those few days, we hoped the patient's own heart would recover sufficiently so that the animal's assist heart could be removed.

My first opportunity to test this new approach presented itself in November 1974, when I operated on a young woman who had previously had an artificial heart valve inserted into the root of the aorta—the main vessel that leads away from the heart to the body.

Because of underdevelopment of this region, the surgeon had only been able to put in the smallest valve available. The patient recovered well from the operation, but she was left with a severe obstruction to the outflow of the left pumping chamber. This resulted in serious symptoms of left heart failure, with breathlessness day and night and the coughing up of frothy sputum and sometimes blood.

Our surgical team decided to operate again to enlarge this area of the heart with a plastic patch so that a larger valve could be inserted.

The operation was completed without any technical problems, but when support from the heart-lung machine was discontinued, the heart failed. Repeated attempts at assisting the heart with the machine and the use of drugs to strengthen the contractions were of no avail, nor was a mechanical assist device connected to the circulation.

At that stage I had the choice of stopping the heart-lung machine and allowing the patient to die or trying the heart of a baboon which I had available. I asked a member of the team to leave the operating room, to explain the problem to the waiting husband and ask his permission for the operation. The husband agreed that we should give his wife that last chance.

The baboon was put to sleep in the laboratory; his heart was removed, brought to the operating room, and placed next to the patient's heart in the piggyback fashion. As soon as the circulation of the baboon heart was restored, it started to beat, sharing the circulatory load to such an extent that we could stop the heart-lung machine.

The operation was completed and the patient returned to the intensive care unit.

Three hours later, however, the baboon heart began to fail, and within half an hour had stopped beating. Although the patient's own heart continued to beat, it had not recovered sufficiently to carry the full circulation, and the patient died.

A few months later, under similar circumstances with a middle-aged man, I used the heart of a chimpanzee. Again, the heart of the ape assisted that of the patient to such an extent that the heart-lung machine could be stopped and the patient returned to the intensive care unit.

The chimpanzee heart continued to function for three days before it showed signs of failure and then stopped. Unfortunately, the patient's heart at that stage had not yet recovered enough to carry the full load, and he died shortly thereafter.

Autopsies in both patients revealed that we had not been able to control the immunological damage to the primate hearts, and both had stopped functioning because of severe rejection.

I decided to abandon the use of animal hearts—the baboon because of the acuteness of rejection and the chimpanzee for a much different reason.

When I first decided on the project, I had bought two male chimps from a primate colony in Holland—The Netherlands. They lived next to each other in separate cages for several months before I used one as a donor.

When we put him to sleep in his cage in preparation for the operation, he chattered and cried incessantly. We attached no significance to this, but it must have made a great impression on his companion, for when we removed the body to the operating room, the other chimp wept bitterly and was inconsolable for days.

The incident made a deep impression on me. I vowed never again to experiment with such sensitive creatures—although I still believe that use of the chimpanzee heart with different methods of immunological suppression would be a workable method of heart assist.

I donated the surviving chimp to an animal farm not far from Cape Town where he met a female mate. The couple have since had their first baby.

Today, the heart from a human donor connected in the piggyback fashion is the only means whereby a totally implanted device can assist the human heart for any length of time. And the procedure came about because I was challenged to find a way to give a terminally ill patient one more chance.

──────Six──────

The concept of "death with dignity" has become an increasing focus of debate, not the least because of medical progress that has brought about demographic changes in population and a major increase in the number of retired and aged persons. The issue has generated a welter of legislation, much of which confuses rather than clarifies a salient question in euthanasia: Who will pull the plug?

Possibly one of the more useful outlines of the problem was put forward by Dr. Joseph Fletcher, a professor of medical ethics at the University of Virginia, in a paper given at a 1974 Euthanasia Conference in New York.

He listed eight levels of attitude and opinion on the human initiatives that can be exercised in the case of a patient dying of an incurable disease.

These are as follows:

1. An absolute refusal to elicit any human initiative in the death or the dying. Life must always be considered as the ultimate human value.

63

2. A qualified refusal, in that the doctor can refrain from employing *extraordinary means* of preserving life but would nevertheless do whatever possible by ordinary means to keep life going.

3. Declining to start treatment in a patient who has an incurable disease and is suffering from a curable inter-current illness (for example, the terminally ill cancer patient with pneumonia). The doctor refuses to initiate treatment for the lung infection that can be cured and in this way may actually hasten death.

4. Stoppage of treatment, with consent, where it is the patient's wish not to be treated any further.

5. Stoppage of treatment, without consent, when the attending physician feels that further treatment can only prolong suffering.

6. Leaving the patient with an overdose of narcotic or sedative, thus assisting the dying person to take his own life.

7. Prior permission is given by the patient to the doctor to administer an injection, under certain circumstances, from which the patient will not recover.

8. Without consent, and on his own authority, the doctor ends the patient's life with an overdose of drugs.

It is clear that the second, third, fourth, and fifth situations are gradations of passive euthanasia. In none of these does the doctor take the initiative in ending the patient's life. The sixth, seventh, and eighth describe grades of active participation.

There is thus a distinct difference between passive—or indirect—euthanasia, where death is induced by suspension of treatment, and the so-called active or direct euthanasia, where death is brought about by a definite act.

To give you an idea of how complex the issue has become, a question has been raised as to the effect a person's decision to "die with dignity" might have on death benefits and estate planning.

An article in the American *Journal of Taxation* cites the hypothetical case of an individual kept alive by mechanical means who chooses to discontinue life support. If that decision is considered an act of suicide, the article says, it could affect insurance policy proceeds. Furthermore, the discussion continues, election to end one's own life could also affect such estate-planning considerations as the timing of realization of income, the gift-tax election, and the year of death choice.

In general, the layman's view of euthanasia is one of "mercy killing," or active intervention to end life, with little or no concept of the possibility of a passive form.

I once visited Perth, Australia, for the purpose of appearing on a marathon round-the-clock television program to raise funds for the treatment of sick children. On a radio program on the day before my television appearance I told an interviewer that I believed doctors were not put on this earth to conquer death and that when a patient was terminally ill with an incurable disease he or she should be allowed to die in peace and comfort.

There was an immediate telephone call from a very upset mother who said my statement had disqualified me from appearing on a television program in aid of sick children. She said, "I am very glad you had not attended me during the birth of my last child because you would probably have killed the child when you saw that it was born a cripple."

I make no excuses and ask no forgiveness for admitting that I have practiced passive euthanasia for many years. In fact, I gave instructions to the doctor attending my own mother in her last illness that she should receive no antibiotics nor be tube fed. At that stage, she was in her ninety-eighth year, suffering from her third stroke and unconscious with pneumonia.

I am convinced that is what she wanted. During the eleven years after her first stroke, as she lay bed-ridden with repeated bladder and lung infections, she told me on occasion, "I wish God would come and take me away."

Before she lapsed into unconsciousness after her last seizure, she repeated over and over again, "Thank you very much, thank you very much."

Those words puzzled me for months after her death, but I am now convinced that she knew the end was near and was expressing her thanks that her long suffering was coming to an end. *The physician who wrote this book states:*

I have never practiced *active* euthanasia, a deed that in my country is regarded as murder and could merit the death penalty. But I do believe that in the clinical practice of medicine, active euthanasia has a definite place. I also believe that we should not be afraid to discuss its place in the scheme of things and to explore the possibilities in this approach to the terminally ill.

I cannot accept the simple statement that a doctor does not have the right to take life, and, as I've already pointed out, the greatest difficulty is to define life.

As a scientist and a humanitarian, I find society's attitude toward the different ways of causing the death of an individual both hypocritical and illogical. Consider that, for as long as man has inhabited the earth, he has accepted with few reservations the right to kill and be killed on the battlefield, even when this leads to not only his own but multiple deaths.

The decision to enter into such mass killing is usually taken by a country's rulers. The individual, as such, has little say in the matter, and not infrequently the reasons given for killing total strangers are seldom clear to those compelled to kill.

Illogicality is compounded by the fact that it is not the aged, the crippled, and the socially defective who are selected to kill and be killed, but the very flower of the country's youth—the young and the healthy.

Refusal to accept battle training can result in a jail sentence. Refusal to kill on the battlefield can earn a court-martial and, in some cases, a death sentence.

The whole process of mass killing between opposing groups is carried out with great patriotic fervor, the trained killer being sent off to the sound of martial music and waving flags. And with great pride, the death toll of the opposing group is headlined in the daily newspapers.

The trained killer who kills more than others is often decorated for his courage and skill in achieving what is seen as something meritorious, and a hero's welcome awaits him when he returns home.

In most countries the so-called defense budget

overshadows the amount allocated to maintaining health and welfare. Vast sums are spent on research projects to make weapons that can kill faster and more efficiently than previous models.

In such situations, society gives healthy young men and women the right to kill other healthy young people whom they have never met—and throughout history this has been done on a scale that has brought untold suffering and loss to millions. Yet the pursuit of such mindless slaughter is often seen as a worthwhile career for intelligent youth.

But what an outcry of horror is heard when a doctor asks for the right to actively end the suffering of a terminally ill patient.

In my own country, and in many other civilized countries, we accept the right of a judge to condemn another human being to death for a capital offense and to request the government to carry out the sentence. Great care is taken that such a death is quick and clean.

Yet what a furor when someone suggests giving the dying patient a similar right to a quick, clean death.

In the past ten years the demand for more liberal abortion laws has resulted in a human wave of aborted fetuses. Thousands of lives are almost literally washed down the drain.

But consider what happens when there is a request for the right to terminate a life that has lost all quality.

As I have pointed out, passive euthanasia is accepted in general by the medical profession, the major religions, and society at large. Therefore, when it is permissible for treatment to be stopped or not instituted to allow the patient to die, it makes for small mercy and less sense when the next logical step—of actively terminating life and hence suffering—is not taken. Why, at that point, can life not be brought to an end instead of extending the suffering of the patient by hours or days or even weeks?

There is also the extension of mental and physical trauma to the loved ones to consider and, not least of all, the extended stay in a hospital that may put a family into a financial plight.

It seems clear to me that a deliberate act of omission, when death is the goal or purpose sought, is morally indistinguishable from a deliberate act of commission. Procedurally, there is a difference between direct and indirect euthanasia, but ethically they are the same.

I have talked to legal, ethical, and medical authorities in many parts of the world on the need for active euthanasia, the problems that would confront the doctor in such situations, and the safeguards required. Again and again the same questions came up:

Who will decide when a life is to be terminated and how can mistakes be avoided?

Would doctors perhaps misuse the right to take life by getting rid of the people they do not like?

Would the medical profession not lose a lot of the trust that is placed in it if doctors were given the right to take life?

Does a doctor have the right to play God?

Must God be the final arbiter on the taking of life?

If it is feared that a doctor is playing God when he terminates a life, it can just as readily be argued that he is playing the same role when he prolongs the life of a terminally ill patient. And surely, when the terminally ill person develops an intercurrent infection that will cause death if not treated, are we not also interfering with God's will by instituting treatment and preventing the patient from dying of the infection?

Generally, these same questions can be raised about war, capital punishment, and abortion. I maintain that if doctors are given the right to practice active euthanasia, and all the necessary safeguards are developed, then most of these objections would fall away.

And at the risk of finding myself out on a theological limb, I say that if it is playing God to reduce human suffering, then I do not believe that the God of mercy and compassion would mind if we mere mortals play God under such circumstances. When we glibly bracket talk of terminating life with mention of the Deity, what in fact do we know of God's interpretation of life?

Is it mere presence of the beating heart and respiratory movements, or is it something more complex? I have not the faintest doubt that when God created man in His own image and breathed life into him, He had a different concept of the meaning of life than the drug-saturated, pain-crazed patient who may not feel the pain but feels no contact with reality either, or the thrashing around on a sweat-soaked bed of a body whose mind is darkened in agony, its only reaction being the purely animal one of trying to escape pain.

The danger is always present that any right should not be granted, but rather that more stringent controls be enforced.

For example, the doctor has the right to diagnose death, but there have been cases of people being buried alive in error; the doctor has the right to remove a diseased organ, such as a lung or kidney, yet legal case studies abound of instances where normal lungs or kidneys were removed.

Such errors are rarely made when proper control is insisted upon. For instance, in recognized medical institutions, important decisions involving care of a patient are never made by one doctor but by a team of qualified persons and usually after consultation with relatives.

When I was a young doctor, serving a residency in obstetrics and gynecology, I often saw patients with cancer of the cervix and uterus. In the advanced form, the condition may invade the nerves at the back of the womb and cause great pain.

Maria was one such patient. Her cervical cancer was too advanced for surgical treatment. At certain times, usually at night, she suffered the most unbelievable agony. Often when I was on overnight duty I sat by her bedside trying to comfort her as she wept and called on God to put her out of her pain.

Drugs gave her only a brief respite. It was a situation that forced me to rely on the bewildering array of textbook knowledge and limited experience at my command. The words of one of my teachers flashed through my mind: "If no cure is available, the doctor is required to alleviate pain and suffering as much as possible."

For the supreme relief of supreme suffering, there is only one answer. I remember that I went about it quite calmly, in complete control of my feelings, going deliberately to the drug cupboard and taking twelve tablets from a bottle marked Morphia gr.¼. One tablet would have been a normal dose to provide pain relief for a woman patient.

In the stillness of the night I found that I handled the preparations with the kind of confidence usually found in someone of far greater experience than I. In those days morphine for injection had to be mixed in a teaspoon of distilled water and held over a flame until dissolved. I made up the solution and went back to Maria's room.

She was quiet when I came to her with the syringe. She looked up at me without a sound, a trusting look in her dark pain-filled eyes.

I found that I could not give her the injection. The will to do so had deserted me. She was like an innocent lamb, waiting for slaughter. Inserting the needle would have been like putting a knife to her throat.

I turned, walked to a sink, and squirted out the morphine solution. In the wardroom a few minutes later I put my face against the wall and felt the veins pounding in my head. I was shaking in the sudden release from stress; it was an overwhelmingly emotional experience.

Two or three weeks later, I saw my patient leave the hospital—her husband's arm around her and two children tugging on her robe. With the help of radium therapy, she had made a remarkable temporary recovery.

There is no doubt Maria had terminal cancer. But, as so often happens with this, the most dreaded of

diseases, there was a period of remission which ena-
bled her to spend a little more time with her loved
ones.

Those who would argue against the system of
active medical euthanasia may well claim, "You see,
that is the danger. You have shown that mistakes can
be made."

The truth is that such a case is the exception.
What was lacking at that point in my life (and for that
matter is still lacking) was proper direction—
guidelines for a physician to follow when confronted
with such a vital medical dilemma.

Among the principles I would like to see governing the practice of medical euthanasia is the rule
that no single doctor should be required to make the
decision alone.

Certainly not a physician only three months
into his residency.

For centuries, society has placed trust in the
medical profession to *help actively* the patient to recover
from ill health. It is simply an extension of this trust to
permit the doctor to actively help the patient in the
process of dying.

One of the major areas of confusion surrounding this very sensitive issue is that it is seldom the
qualified person who pronounces judgment or pur-
ports to speak with authority on the problem.

By way of example, in the early days after the
first human heart transplant I was often asked,
"Would you like to have your heart transplanted?" My
answer was that of course I would not like to have my
heart transplanted, just as I would not like to have a leg

amputated or undergo any other major form of surgery.

But, as I pointed out, they were asking the wrong person. My wishes would be different if I were dying from extensive destruction of the heart muscle and the only operation that could help was a heart transplant; or if I were suffering from extensive gangrene of the foot and my days and nights were spent in agony.

That is why I say that most of those who insist that a doctor should not actively help a patient end the distress of dying are not qualified. They are disqualified by reason of their noninvolvement. The relevant opinion is that of the dying person, or the relatives who know what the patient's requirements are or have watched their loved one's prolonged suffering.

In South Africa there was a widely publicized case of a young doctor who gave his aged and injured father a drug overdose because, in his view, that was the best treatment for the old man.

The father was a terminal patient suffering from cancer of the prostate, a disease that often disseminates to the bone and causes intense pain.

At first the doctor had tried to alleviate his father's suffering by using morphine and other painkilling drugs. After a time, even this became ineffective and the young man was forced to watch in anguish as day after day, in reaction to the cancer spreading through his body, his father lay racked with pain.

Also unhappy at the quality of nursing the old man was receiving in the small rural hospital to which he had been admitted, the son's compassion at last overcame the ethical restraint he had learned as a doctor. He gave his father an overdose of intravenous anesthetic.

Immediately a look of calm came over the old man's face as he fell off to sleep and died.

Legally, it was an open-and-shut case. The doctor had performed active euthanasia on a patient. He had taken a life.

The civil court in South Africa found him guilty of murder. The twist is that the judge was in complete sympathy with the actions of the doctor. He found extenuating circumstances in the fact that the accused had been a loving son who had become emotionally overwrought by his father's sufferings.

Considering the current dogmatic attitude toward euthanasia, it was quite a revelation to see how leniently the judiciary viewed this crime. When the young doctor was found guilty, he was sentenced to be detained until the "rising of the court," which meant that he was free to go as soon as the judge had left the room.

But what a different picture it was when the doctor had to face his peers, his colleagues in the medical profession. In South Africa all doctors found guilty of civil or criminal offenses are automatically tried again by a sitting of the profession's disciplinary body.

The Medical Council found the doctor guilty of malpractice. Not murder—malpractice. And the jury of doctors was much more severe than the civil court. The accused was stripped of his license to practice medicine. It was several years before he was allowed to resume work as a doctor.

The question of who was right opens whole

vistas of medical ethics, bounded by necessity and that cool, clear, and most pure of human responses—mercy.

Possibly the argument itself is a category mistake, a failure to use the right language in describing the problem. As soon as we speak of right and wrong in a particular context, we are forced to choose sides.

Only in the very narrowest sense, constrained perhaps by a strict legal or ethical code that brooks no definition of a situation other than the official view laid down by the rule book, is it possible to pronounce judgment.

That, of course, was the situation to which both the judicial and medical disciplinary processes were committed. Both were created for and served society at large and, in so doing, inevitably became institutionalized.

As far as the court was concerned, the doctor had committed a crime—but under extenuating circumstances. The judge weighed the facts and found that justice would be served through leniency.

The Medical Council took the view that boundaries had not been drawn for the practice of active euthanasia. They felt that the doctor had practiced medicine in a way unacceptable to society—or at least to society at that moment in time. Punishment was indicated to set an example for the rest of the profession.

The Council's action was intended as a deterrent to other doctors, to make them realize that in medicine, active euthanasia cannot be acceptable in one instance and not in another—at least not until

76

Once again, the author reiterates—

there are safeguards against misuse of death-promoting medical treatment.

I have never practiced active euthanasia, for one reason only—it is illegal. But I have often stood at the bedside of a dying patient and realized the need for this service.

Those who claim that one can always alleviate the suffering of the dying has either not had enough exposure to the problem or is lacking in a simple quality—compassion.

─── Seven ───

Sometimes I think that society places too much responsibility on mere mortals who have been trained in the healing arts. A physician can diagnose and treat illness—yes, even postpone death—but he cannot prevent life from ending when the time has come.

At times a family can become so emotionally involved when a loved one is critically ill that the doctor in attendance is subjected to unbelievable pressures.

I remember an incident from many years ago when I was in general practice in a country town in South Africa. I was called to a farm, arriving at the little whitewashed house with its tin roof just as the sun was going down. As I got out of my car, the peace and tranquillity of the countryside overwhelmed me.

On a South African farm the end of the day is such a special time. The cows were coming back from the fields; the chickens were being fed; the ducks and geese were scurrying in all directions.

In the midst of all the activity, I noticed a goat

tethered to a stake near the front porch of the farmhouse. I assumed he was there to be milked. He bleated as though to call my attention to his discomfort.

Before I had time to knock, an anxious-looking elderly woman opened the door and immediately escorted me to the bedroom where her husband was lying. He had high fever with a rapid pulse rate. With each breath, his nostrils would dilate widely to allow as much air as possible to reach his lungs. Pneumonia was indicated, and on examining his chest, my fears were confirmed. Almost three-quarters of the right lung was solid with inflammation.

There was no doubt that the patient was seriously ill with lumbar pneumonia. This was in the days before antibiotics were freely available, and there was little I could do. Treatment of pneumonia then consisted mainly of treating the symptoms and waiting until the patient's own resistance overcame the infection.

In pre-antibiotic days, the clinical condition of patients suffering from lumbar pneumonia (usually caused by pneumococcus) followed a typical course. The patient's condition would worsen until the seventh or eleventh day, when what was called the crisis set in, and the patient either recovered or his condition became extreme and death intervened.

When my examination of the farmer was completed, it was apparent that the course of the disease would be determined in the next few hours. I decided to stay on the farm that night and minister to him as best I could.

In the early hours of the morning, the farmer's

condition deteriorated. He became delirious, his fever rose, and his pulse weakened. His wife knew, as I did, that the crisis was near.

She called me to the kitchen to have a cup of coffee. Suddenly she said, "Dr. Barnard, have you done everything you can to save my husband's life?"

"Yes," I replied, "I've tried everything."

She looked at me, tears welling in her eyes. Her voice was almost a whisper. "We haven't tried heat. My parents said that was the most helpful in any kind of inflammation."

"How do you propose to apply heat to the chest?" I asked.

"Well, the old 'farmer's remedy' was to kill an animal, skin him quickly, and wrap the warm skin around the chest of the sick person, so that the heat penetrated to the lungs."

I struggled not to show my feelings. I was young and naïve, and I felt it would be a disgrace to the medical profession if, after studying for so many years, I had to go out in the dark and kill an animal just to get its skin to treat my patient.

"It's three o'clock now. Let's wait a little longer—until half-past five—before we try a farm remedy."

Almost lost in her misery and her urgent need to do something for the man she loved, she could do little but agree.

At five o'clock I examined my patient and found to my relief that his temperature had gone down and he was resting more comfortably. The crisis was over, and there was no doubt he would recover.

An hour later he was much better. I chatted

briefly with his wife about further treatment, assured her that I would keep in touch, and walked out onto the front porch of the farmhouse.

The sun had risen and the farmyard was a busy hive of animal activity. It was truly exhilarating to see the early morning surge of life and smell the many smells that go to make up a farm.

The goat was still tethered to the stake in the yard. "Goat," I said, half aloud, "I suppose you know I saved your life."

Its answer was a plaintive bleat.

I grinned all the way to my car before it suddenly struck me—the goat's life was the only one I'd saved.

The concern of that rural South African housewife, her willingness to resort to any end to keep her husband alive, shows how emotionally involved a family can become when a loved one is critically ill.

The involvement can, of course, take other forms. It need not be a last-ditch stand. Sometimes sympathy for an incurable family member turns to compassion, and death is looked on as a savior.

In the summer of 1975, the name Karen Quinlan burst on the news scene. To physicians throughout the world, it was an old story. The parents of a twenty-one-year-old girl in Morris County, New Jersey, were distraught to see their daughter in a coma for four months—victim of a mysterious disease that had caused massive cerebral damage.

Doctors said there was no hope of recovery, but—in conforming with accepted medical practice—she was kept on a respirator to sustain her breathing and blood circulation.

If it meant that she would eke out an existence without any kind of meaning, the parents, Mr. and Mrs. Joseph T. Quinlan, saw no reason to use mechanical life-sustaining procedures on their daughter. They asked doctors to turn the respirator off, or, as the colloquial expression so popular in the media had it, to "pull the plug."

My memory of the Quinlan case is especially vivid because, at the time, I had been invited to the United States by several medical societies to tell about the new "twin heart" transplant procedure.

In the cities that I visited, my host physicians asked me to appear on local and network radio and television programs. With few exceptions, the interviewers asked my opinion of the medical dilemma going on in Morris County.

Perhaps a sociologist who is experienced in researching the effects of so-called media events on the general public can explain why this isolated incident in a quiet New York City suburb had such a worldwide effect on the ethical and legal ground rules of the medical profession.

The problem posed by that young woman as she lay breathing mechanically day after day in a fixed death-in-life situation sparked new discussions on the definition of death. It set a legal precedent for future court actions and laid the groundwork for passage of legislation granting terminally ill persons and their families the right to authorize withdrawal of life-sustaining procedures when death was believed imminent.

Perhaps it could even be said that I would not now be presenting my own case for medical euthanasia if Karen Quinlan's plight had not focused the world's attention on the subject.

But the Quinlan situation was not uncommon in clinical medicine. There can be few doctors who in treating critically ill patients have not faced a similar dilemma: a loved one, unconscious for an extended length of time; a team of doctors determined to abide by ethical and legal ground rules, and a family who begs, "Please, please—let God take her and put an end to the suffering."

Each doctor handles these emotionally charged incidents in the way the situation determines—that is part of the practice of medicine. But it is clear that the salient question in all cases is: to treat or not to treat; to continue prolongation of life through artificial means or to withdraw treatment already instituted in order to shorten the process of dying.

In certain cases the dilemma goes further. The doctor has to decide whether to give the necessary drugs in sufficient doses to alleviate the distressing symptoms that may be present in the dying patient when there is the risk that the drugs may contribute to the patient's death.

On occasion I, and many of my colleagues, have decided to fight to the bitter end. And with modern technology, the end can often be long in coming, delayed in some cases for weeks or months.

When Louis Washkansky, my first heart transplant patient, was suffocating to death from widespread infection, with no hope of cure, I seriously contemplated the possibility of connecting him to an artificial oxygenator so that he could survive another one or two days.

When Dr. Philip Blaiberg, the second patient to receive a transplanted human heart, survived eighteen months after the operation and then became severely debilitated from extensive drug treatment and chronic rejection, I was madly looking for a donor so that I could transplant a second heart into his body. In times of crisis, you grasp at straws.

In each instance, I was persuaded by a much wiser colleague, the late Professor Val Schrire, not to go ahead but rather to do everything possible to make the patient comfortable while dying.

I can relate many more such experiences, as no doubt can any other doctor, of times when I struggled for days to keep a patient "alive" when there was no hope at all. At such times, when the patient eventually died, I felt let down and often blamed the other members of my team for not pulling their weight.

I would lie awake at night and relive those moments of defeat, searching for ways and means by which to beat death. The next morning I would get out of bed in a state of depression, unwilling to face the day because I had lost.

Why did I behave in that way? Why do doctors insist on using heroic means to delay death in the presence of incurable, terminal disease? These questions concern me more and more.

What is clear is that there is undue emphasis in the education of the young doctor and, in later years, an incorrect concept of what is meant by good surgical and medical results.

The doctor is taught to see himself as a champion chosen for one purpose only—the preservation of life. In practice, results are in the main judged solely on survival rates. In an almost insidious way, he is led to see the sole aim of his skills as directed to the prevention of death. When he reads a paper to his peers at a medical meeting, the question of results is often presented as a victory over death or illness: So many patients survived for such and such a length of time. But little, if any, emphasis is given to what sort of life the patients had as a result of the treatments.

The undue emphasis placed on the conquering of death became apparent to me after the first heart transplant. In tours and lectures in many parts of the world, whether speaking to my peers or to laymen, I was confronted with the same question: How long did your patient live after the transplant?

Surely the better question would have been: *How* did your patient live after the transplant?

The inclination to judge medical achievement on the basis of survival statistics severely harmed the heart transplant program. In both the medical and lay press the deaths of transplant patients and the lengths of their survival were highlighted as news. Little, if anything, was said about the improved quality of life for those patients, even though they lived only a month or a few years after the operation.

I remember a journalist asking Dr. Blaiberg, the first heart transplant patient to have recovered sufficiently to leave the hospital, when he first decided that the operation was a success.

"As soon as I woke up and drew my first breath," was Dr. Blaiberg's reply. He explained that when he realized he could breathe freely again and did not have to gasp and fight for each lungful of air, he knew the operation had been a success. It had immediately improved the quality of his life.

In some countries, where lawsuits against doctors for negligence and malpractice are a favorite pastime, the fear of litigation can be counterproductive to good medical practice. Who can say to what extent it influences the choice of "safe" treatment that is of no value at all in place of a more effective course of action that might lay the medical practitioner open to legal claims.

I have mentioned the reason why the first heart transplant was carried out in South Africa (i.e., elsewhere it could only be done in an acute situation where the patient could not be weaned from the heart-lung machine and where a donor was coincidentally available). This conclusion was paramount because surgeons in other countries were afraid that if the operation were carried out under any other preconditions and was unsuccessful they would lay themselves open to suit for malpractice or negligence.

This situation is feared less in South Africa, where there is quite a different legal approach to medical malpractice and negligence. There the standard of medicine is stringently controlled by the South African Medical and Dental Council, and civil suits against doctors are uncommon. Under such circumstances, there was of course a much greater professional risk of doing the operation.

There is no doubt that a doctor's behavior and actions must be controlled, but it is better for the public if this control is exerted mainly by his peers and not by the courts.

Medical technology has developed to such an extent in the past twenty-five years that its very effectiveness has given us previously unconsidered ethical problems, particularly in relation to the treatment of the terminally ill.

At the 1971 Annual Health Conference of the New York Academy of Medicine, Lord Ritchie-Calder summed it up correctly when he said, "Medical science has produced an ethical crisis which transcends our conventional ideas of good and evil."

In a strikingly written pamphlet distributed by the Euthanasia Council in New York, Dr. Nancy I. Caroline relates the beautiful story of Eli Kahn. Admitted to the hospital at the age of seventy-eight, his condition is described in his own words: "The engine is broken down, it is time for the engineer to abandon it."

In spite of repeated requests to leave him alone so that he could die with dignity, medical treatment was instituted and increased until eventually he was intubated and connected to a mechanical respirator.

That night he woke up, reached over and switched off the ventilator, and died. But before he lost consciousness he had time to scrawl a message to his physician. It read, "Death is not the enemy, doctor. Inhumanity is."

I hold that the patient knows what is humane and what is relevant in his situation. What role then can society play in preventing the kind of inhumanity that occurs every day in large hospitals, where patients are treated, not to alleviate their suffering, but often because doctors want to try out their mastery of death-delaying techniques?

Society can ask for three things: that doctors be humanitarians and not merely scientists; that life-support mechanisms and other aspects of modern medical technology not be used where there is no hope; and that when the patient is suffering from severe pain it be relieved by medicines even if this means shortening the life of the patient.

This, in my opinion, is what is meant by passive euthanasia—and that is why I have pleaded in my own country for full support for such an approach. It allows the medical staff to give the terminally ill a comfortable, dignified death. A doctor who holds such a viewpoint is not trying to kill his patients; rather he believes they have the right to die in comfort.

The question then arises: Are we not playing God, making ourselves the arbiters of life and death?

My reply is also a question: Have we not perverted the Christian tradition into the belief that biological existence per se is of supreme value and, on the basis of that interpretation, sidetracked ourselves into an ethical dilemma of ghastly proportions?

The obvious error is that we mistake mere biological existence for life and that we believe it to be of supreme importance to continue such life, even in a human being condemned through illness to a vegetative state. In such cases, is it not more Christian or more Godly to allow nature to take its course? That is really all that passive euthanasia requires.

Let us see how religion views passive euthanasia. I would have expected, for example, that those most opposed to it would be Orthodox Jews. I have conferred with Rabbi Immanuel Jacobowitz and have read his book on medical ethics, written in 1959.

The Orthodox Jewish view accepts the legality of expediating the death of an incurably ill patient in acute agony by withholding such medicaments as would sustain his continued existence by "unnatural means." In such teaching there is nothing opposed to passive euthanasia, merely agreement that no special treatment should be used to continue a life that is already at an end.

In 1950, the Roman Catholic view was clearly stated by Pope Pius XII in a series of addresses on medical ethics. He pointed out that there was no absolute obligation on the part of the physician to employ extraordinary means to preserve life. These he defined as means that cannot be obtained without undue expense, pain, or other inconvenience and that give no reasonable hope of providing benefit.

I have not seen a really authoritative Protestant statement, but from what I have read on the subject there appears to be general agreement that life should not simply be preserved merely because it is medically feasible to do so.

Islamic attitudes are based on the Koran, which holds that death is beyond the control of all but Allah and prescribes severe punishment for those who violate the sanctity of life. Salman Navdi, professor of Islamic studies at the University of Durban-Westville, told a symposium on euthanasia that pulling the plug on a patient may be permissible "with lots of ifs and buts" and only perhaps in an extreme situation— such as when the choice is limited between postponing death in a terminal case and use of the machine for another patient with better chance of survival.

The Hindu stand is clear: Euthanasia in any form has no place in the Hindu scriptures. According to Dr. T. P. Mishra, an expert in Sanskrit at the Durban University, it is "clearly stated that the soul has to undergo all pleasures and pains allotted to a body in which it resides."

Buddhists consider human life to be meaningful only when the higher cognitive, sapient faculties are capable of being exercised. They would like to see death defined as that state in which the patient has ceased to exist as a person, which generally occurs upon irreversible failure of the cerebrum.

Above all, Buddhists maintain that it is as immoral to inflict unwarranted pain and suffering on an ill and dying person as it is on a healthy one. They consider life to be precious but not sacred or divine. In their scheme of things, there are no souls that can be "saved" or "lost" or "returned" to their Maker.

I am struck by the fact that an overall view of religious conviction on the subject gives the impression that the various churches are more willing to accept the aims of euthanasia than the medical profession, and that euthanasia is more in keeping with religious teaching than it is with medical teaching.

Generally, the supreme value in our religious heritage is placed on the personhood of man, the person in his wholeness, his freedom, his integrity, and dignity. When illness brings a person to a state in which he is less than free, and less able to sustain his dignity and integrity, then what is most precious is gone.

The obvious conclusion is that, when personhood is gone, mere continuation of existence by means of artificial life support is a violation of an individual's right.

What better argument is there in favor of society's acceptance of the use of euthanasia?

Eight

The suffering of children is one of the most heartbreaking of hospital problems. Their innocence and total trust in nurses and doctors makes it even more poignant, especially when the outcome offers little hope.

It has been my experience that the doctor-patient relationship with a child is as rewarding for the doctor, if not more so, as it is for the child. It was out of a multiplicity of such relationships that I was able to formulate a personal view of what good quality of life should be.

Let me explain.

Children will undergo the most mutilating surgery, secure in the knowledge that the hospital staff will put it right—that in the end, life will be as good as that enjoyed by other children. It is a ruling philosophy among child patients. But heaven help the doctor who shows lack of confidence.

An Italian boy thought I was some kind of god

when I first examined him. His confidence in me shone like a ray of light. After a major heart operation, he seemed to make a good recovery, and then complications set in.

He was a brave kid. He fought hard—until the day I allowed my doubts to show during an examination.

He smiled at me. I frowned back. I was too concerned about his condition to return his smile, and I probably also communicated some of my anxiety in my voice as I spoke to the nurse. I was a worried man, and I looked it.

His condition worsened from then on, and that night he turned his face to the wall and died.

By contrast, another child was a different case. Karen—as we will call her—was seven years old. She had a single ventricle and a single atrium—a heart of two chambers instead of the normal four. Colleagues advised that it would be foolish to tackle such a difficult case, to try to reconstruct such an anomaly.

I must say that I was tempted to agree. This was at a time when I had the feeling that the press was watching over my shoulder as I operated. Reporters were phoning my office daily. Whatever I did was regarded as worth reporting.

And if a child were to be brought to Cape Town from her home a long distance away only to die after an operation, it was a foregone conclusion that the next day's headlines would call me a butcher.

But I've always believed that fear of personal consequences should be the least of the criteria to consider in surgery. The patient's wants are always a primary consideration. I went to visit Karen.

She had blue eyes, a rosebud mouth, and a lilt in her voice that tugged at the heartstrings.

"What's wrong with you, love," I asked her. She looked up and answered with a smile that melted my pretense of an unemotional facade.

"I have a broken heart."

That did it. I'm not ashamed to say that I left the room with tears in my eyes and a determination to do what I could for the child even if her case appeared hopeless.

The idea of failure went out of the window. Surgery was scheduled as quickly as possible, and the next time I saw the child with a "broken heart" she was under anesthesia, a look of trust on her face.

When Karen's chest cavity was opened and I had a chance to study her two-chambered heart, I knew my years of training in cardiac surgery were not in vain. I saw what was required to restore the heart's pumping function.

The operation took six hours. At the end of the surgery I knew that we had created a working heart—the broken heart had been repaired. Karen would live to play childhood games again, just as my own daughter had played when she was seven years old.

The total trust of the child patient places a heavy burden on the nursing and medical staff, not only to ensure the best outcome but also to maintain personality growth during the long weeks and months that the child may be in the hospital.

It may be necessary to discipline an afflicted child, and it would indeed be a heart of stone that could bear this duty without some inner misgiving.

I shall never forget the day I saw a "Grand Prix"

held in a children's surgical ward. In the face of pain and mutilation, it was an inspired piece of sheer joy in living.

It happened spontaneously when someone carelessly left a food trolley unattended in a corner of the ward. A moment's inattention by the ward staff, and the trolley was commandeered by an intrepid crew of two—a driver and a mechanic.

The mechanic provided the motive power by galloping along behind, head down, pushing on the rear rail, while the driver squatted on the lower deck of the trolley, clinging on with one hand and steering by scraping one foot on the floor.

The choice of roles was easy: The mechanic was blind and the driver had only one arm.

They put on a hell-on-wheels show that, judging by the yells of encouragement from the rest of the patients, had more spectator appeal than any road or track race.

It ended in a confusion of scattered plates and outraged scolding from the ward sister, who brushed aside explanations of "Gee, sister, we were only practicing for the Granpree" and ordered the offenders back to bed.

The mechanic was all of seven years old. A child from a slum dwelling, he had lost his sight in a sudden blaze that destroyed not only his firetrap home but also most of his face.

He was partway through a weary round of operations to release his jaw from the mass of scar tissue that had gripped it so solidly that he could only raise his head by opening his mouth.

At the time of the "Granpree," he was a walking

horror with a ruined face and a long flap of skin hanging loose from one side of his neck to his body. This was the skin graft with which it was planned to release his head from its fleshy trap and give him some neck movement.

In a previous operation, the graft had been scraped free from an unburned section of his body and rolled into a tube, with one end still attached to maintain blood supply and the other end swung up and grafted onto his neck.

When the graft became firmly enough attached and had developed an alternative blood supply, it would be cut off at the body; the tube would be opened to make a flat skin flap, the scar tissue cut away from under the jaw, and the skin flap placed on top.

If all went well, he would have good neck movement, and most of his terrible scars would be covered. But it would be a long and painful time of being wheeled in and out of operating rooms, of healing wounds and the awful discomfort of heavy bandaging.

"We won," he told me, appearing from under the bedclothes minutes after ward discipline had been restored and sister's awful threats of punishment were still hanging in the air.

His sunken eye sockets focused on me in the uncanny way of the blind, and his head bobbed up and down.

The mechanic was laughing.

The driver was nine. The full book of troubles had been thrown at him by the time he was seven—beginning with an illness-ridden infancy, an operation for the correction of a faulty heart valve (with an amazing recovery), polio and the loss of leg action, broken bones, and recently an operation to remove his right arm and shoulder because of bone cancer.

He explained that the Grand Prix crash was due to mechanical failure owing to the fact that his machine was "just an ole crap trolley" and the wheels too stiff to steer properly.

As I left the ward, he was trading insults with his mechanic.

Filled with pity and some degree of social guilt for these terribly maimed children, I had not gone a hundred paces before it struck me like a hammer blow. Here were two of the most socially deprived people I'd ever met, and they had just given me a lesson in getting on with the business of living.

Since then I've often thought of that incident. And I am grateful to those two kids for the insight that the business of living is joy, in the real sense of the word. Not simply pleasure, amusement, recreation—shallow words in comparison—but more a celebration of being alive.

And while that celebration goes on, we are truly alive.

Surely that should be one of the criteria in determining the basic conditions for active euthanasia. Where there is no more joy in living, no further hope of joy, and no wish to continue, then there can be little problem in arriving at a decision.

The physical condition of the body should never be a deciding factor unless the patient is deeply unconscious and incapable of presenting other criteria. In the case of the maimed children, their joy in living surpassed all physical disabilities.

But without that quality of life, even the physically sound are but moving corpses, though I hesitate to be so dualistic as to describe a suicidally depressed person as physically sound.

Take the situation of grossly or seriously defective children. Visit any institution which, for want of a better word, "cares" for such youngsters. There you will find aberrations of nature that exist as purely stimulus-response organisms. Other than reacting to pain, hunger, and comfort or lack of it, they have no conception of the world.

I recall one child whose condition made a strong impression on me and caused me to rethink my stereotyped, straight-out-of-medical-school approach. He was a hydrocephalic, a child with a tiny undeveloped body and a grossly swollen head, his brain cells crushed by the immense pressure in his skull.

The child's head was so big that he could not lift it from the pillow. The sheer immovable weight was a continual cause of bedsores on the back of the head. His hands had been padded to prevent him from injuring himself as he kept picking, rubbing, and striking at the bedsores. Later it became necessary to tie the child's arms to the bedside.

I asked one nurse how long the child had been like that. She was not only a good and kindly soul, she was a devoted Christian and a skilled professional. Without blinking an eye, she said, "About three years."

I remember walking out of that efficiently run institution—with its polished floors and cheery decor and its hierarchy of steady jobs that would remain secure as long as those "patients" were kept alive—and wondering how quickly my experimental animal laboratory would be closed down if I were to run it as a similar pain factory.

A voluntary euthanasia group in the United Kingdom recently received a donation "in memory of the cruel and totally unnecessary suffering endured by Mrs. Isobel Lejeune."

The donation was sent by her daughter, who said that until her mother was eighty-nine she had never suffered other than minor illnesses. She and her husband had lived gentle, obscure lives, undemanding and happy. No violent emotional disturbances, and even their siblings lived long into old age.

Like millions of others, she was just another loving wife and mother who filled her life with repetitive tasks—important only to the people who knew and loved her. Her husband, who also had good health, died within a few hours of the first symptoms of his final illness, about six months before her eighty-ninth birthday.

Mrs. Lejeune's daughter described the subsequent events: "She was sitting watching the birds in the garden when she suddenly collapsed into a coma—and we were sad, but happy that the inevitable end had come so kindly.

"Then came the nightmare. The doctor came, found she was still breathing, although quite unconscious and she was rushed to the hospital where we had to leave her. We went back next day, thinking to find her quietly slipping away.

"But modern technology can be so shortsighted. The doctors found they could force that tired little body to exist. So, obedient to their shortsighted unthinking conditioned behavior, they did so.

"She was more or less unconscious, but never again coherent, or able to recognize us without confusion. She was incontinent; she had to be fed. They could not keep her in bed without bars.

"Meanwhile she fell often. Three times she broke an arm; on one occasion, her hip. Several times we were called to come immediately as she had fallen and was suffering severe bruising.

"To visit her was anguish—to see her sitting, perhaps with an arm in a sling, and the quiet tears running down her pathetic little face, so bewildered and unhappy.

"This situation went on for nearly three years—until just before Christmas even technology had to yield to nature."

The reason the daughter gave for donating money to the euthanasia group was simply stated: "We despise a system that can inflict such mental and physical pain. This experience has changed our whole outlook. We dread to find ourselves in the power of such people. Please continue your efforts for the sake of the dignity of ordinary decent people."

Even in such exasperating circumstances, the Christian church forbids one obvious solution—the taking of one's life—as an offence against God. To do so would be usurping God's prerogative to give and take life. If we were to follow this view to its logical conclusion, then Christianity should forbid the killing of enemy soldiers in battle, and should even frown on medical care that could possibly prolong life and postpone death.

We are well aware that the official Christian churches do not forbid war and that they even allow the appointment of military chaplains and make no public objection to the award of medals for bravery in combat in which men have died. Nor would it be difficult to find examples in which the Church—on both sides of the clash—prayed for a successful outcome.

Further, I could produce endless cases of ministers of religions of all persuasions who have urged prayer for a seriously ill public personage under medical treatment and have included prayers for the doctors—hardly a recognition of the Deity's right to ordain life.

I take no issue with the Church on this point and have merely used the position to illustrate the lack of clarity and consensus on what is admittedly an emotional subject.

In short, I agree with Toynbee's view that the prolongation of life by human action, as well as the cutting short of life by human action, would be an offense against God if it were true that God alone had the right to decree the length of time a human being may live.

Unfortunately, Christian practice is inconsistent with Christian theory. As a generalization, most Christians would agree with attempts to prolong life and would object to taking life.

The issue then becomes a question of what is meant by life. I have defined it as joy in living. Given the absence of this quality, without hope of restitution, the request of the suffering person (if conscious and *compos mentis*), and the satisfaction of other criteria such as good faith on the part of those caring for the person and the completion of legal requirements, there is no ethical reason why active medical euthanasia may not be administered.

The formalities, the checks and balances, and the legal detail are for the bureaucratic mind to formulate.

I have always wondered at the kind of person who would mercifully end the life of a suffering animal yet would hesitate to extend the same privilege to a fellow being. It may be that in all of us there lurks a sense of guilt—and what more guilt-making burden can we assume than that of responsibility for another's death.

The error, perhaps, is one of category—that of regarding squeamishness as mercy.

Nine

If society insists that the doctor has no right to end the life of a dying patient, can it also insist that the patient has no right to end his own life?

Should an individual, sane in mind, be condemned if, after careful assessment and the conclusion that the quality of his life has deteriorated to the point where it has become meaningless to be alive, he takes his life?

I don't think so. I believe it is a fundamental right of any person who is capable of making a clear assessment of his situation to take his own life. It is a right because no one can stop him and no one can punish him for this action.

Politically and socially, categories are more comfortably dealt with than people. Hence it is easier to make decisions for the masses than for the individual. Thus it follows that in society the individual and individual action are gathered together and judged on general rules.

Man's essence lies in his individuality. That he has emerged as something less than human in terms of mass society is inevitable. Nevertheless, it is impossible, and almost a betrayal of our humanity, to judge a life history with the choice of one of two words: right or wrong.

The conscious existence of most people appears dominated by the desire to go on living. In social relations, emphasis is placed on participation with others and the drive to achieve. The wish to live is a firm but personal animation. Coupled with affection for others, it creates consuming interest in the surrounding world. Death is served by opposing tendencies.

For centuries, men have been disquieted by the recurrence of suicide in their midst. Most men have found it not only incomprehensible but also contemptible that some of their fellows should show a willful preference for death, thus disdaining the existence to which others cling with such tenacity. Such persons, it is said, are unbalanced, mentally incapable of appreciating their good fortune in being alive.

There is a curious illogicality in such a concept of sanity. In our society, the belief is firm that human beings are imbued with an eagerness for life and that longings for death play no part in the healthy personality.

Yet many persons seem to court death, finding a strange exuberance in placing themselves in dangerous situations, such as climbing unstable mountain slopes, sailing in flimsy gliding apparatus, roaring down a track in high-speed cars, or exploring the world underwater. Such men, when killed in the course of their dangerous sport, are publicly mourned.

Contrast this with the situation where a man dies by his own deliberate action, a piece of behavior at once shameful and fear inspiring. Often it is regarded as an escape. The malice and indignation expressed by persons who condemn suicide suggest that they scorn anyone who has effected an escape from life—an escape that they themselves eschew only by stern self-discipline.

Christian dogmatism sees suicide as an act that is wrong and should not be condoned under any circumstances. Yet what of the concentration camp inmate who hurls himself against the electrified wire while being herded to the gas chamber? Can it be wrong for the terminally ill cancer patient who, suffering from the side effects of extensive treatment that has led to hair loss and mouth sores, and paraplegia as a result of a collapsed vertebra, opts to take an overdose of barbiturates?

Even if the concept of suicide is not acceptable to most people, I think that the majority of us understand the reasons why the termination of one's own life can—in some cases—be preferable to staying alive.

To some individuals, just the stress of everyday living is enough to make death more attractive. Suicide can be either a logical, planned ritual or the act of a sick mind.

Psychological experts have even come up with professionally accepted explanations for the ghastly mass suicides in Guyana. The triggering elements, they said, were probably fanatical loyalty to a charismatic leader, who told his followers that suicide was a noble act, and a desperate fear that a hostile outside world was closing in on them.

The same elements were no doubt present during the battle for Masada in the first century A.D., when the besieged Jews committed suicide en masse rather than surrender to the attacking Romans.

Though the outcome was the same in each case, it would perhaps be true to say that the interpretation of events differed. The Jews had been under siege for months and could see the Roman army building a causeway from which to launch the final assault on their fortress. The events in Guyana were hardly based on such concrete evidence.

But each group arrived at the same decision: The quality of life had deteriorated to the point where life was not worth living and should be ended. There was also the possibility of secondary gains, such as an afterlife, for having obeyed instructions from a religious leader.

Perhaps those who fear an upsurge of suicide if the action were made more acceptable could bear in mind that at one time in Western society there were strict antisuicide laws coupled with religious restrictions that included such charming practices as the refusal of Christian burial and ridicule of the corpse.

Much of the legal proscription has been repealed, England being the last to comply in 1961. The change in the legal status of suicide has had no effect on the suicide rate, though other factors now appearing as a result of modern social change may be determining forces.

For example, the steady increase in the number of old people in society, coupled with the ability of modern medicine to prolong the life-span, are basic reasons for the current rise of interest in the legalization of voluntary euthanasia.

In 1970, a draft bill permitting euthanasia for persons suffering from terminal illness was thrown out of the British Parliament on the grounds that it represented "suicide by proxy." The main opposition came from religious and medical quarters, particularly from doctors who feared being cast in the role of executioner.

Enough has been written on the causes and typology of suicide to fill a library. Social scientists have evolved statistical, psychological, economic, and other categories and have even elucidated the groups most at risk, such as males, the aged, the single, divorced, or widowed, the childless, the wealthy, those under tension, and the physically and mentally ill.

Factors that seem to militate against suicide are youth, being female, living in a rural area, religious devotion, being married, having children, being poor, and war.

These are generalizations, and anyone can produce exceptions, but the rule seems consistent with what the two crippled children taught me in the surgical ward—where there is joy in living there is need of life.

An apparent anomaly here are the so-called altruistic suicides, those people who seem to have an excessive sense of duty toward the community, such as the monks who burned themselves to death in Vietnam and the dozen or more French students who immolated themselves during the early 1970s.

I doubt whether there is any such animal as altruism. The outward act of apparent selflessness is there, as in the case of an impulsive need to drop a coin into a blind beggar's cup. When examined, that sudden softening begins to look very much like middle-class guilt.

The giving of the coin, usually so small that its economic effect on the pocket is negligible, gives the donor an instant glow, a warm feeling of having somehow or other helped the human race, or at least one of its members. And that's the reward, an almost priceless psychic lift in return for minimal outlay. So what price altruism?

In the case of altruistic suicide, one wonders how strong the impulse to lay down your life would be if you had no possible hope of reward in the form of either posthumous honor or peer approval before death. Even if the suicide were completely anonymous and had made no attempt at identification before death, there remains a complex of human motivation that must surely provide some form of reward.

Yet the stigma against suicide remains. In almost any Western community there is strong pressure against the labeling of a death as suicide. Practically all families will close ranks and blatantly distort the truth to maintain the fiction.

Possibly the main reason for this is guilt—the feeling that if the dead person chose suicide as an alternative to life, it must necessarily be a value judgment on those most closely associated.

Statistical studies show that mental disorder is indicated in one-third of suicides, a point of view rejected by some sociologists who claim that such illness cannot be quantified. They also point out that, although suicide is seen as an abnormal reaction to stress, it is abnormal only in the sense that it is not the choice of the majority of the population.

Existentialists place great importance on despair and the concept of death as determinants of suicide. It is difficult for most people to conceive of nonexistence, hence suicide would be seen as an event in the life of the person who destroys himself.

Other existentialist views reject the idea of suicide prevention as merely a medical prejudice against death. Suicide, they feel, is called for when death is needed by the soul.

Certainly most religions support the concept of an afterlife. Death—whether self-inflicted or not—is often regarded as a new beginning. It would be an unusual person who regarded suicide as total cessation of being.

Comparative psychology has produced no evidence in normal animals—under normal conditions of self-destructive behavior—that could be interpreted as a wish to die, so it would appear that man is the only animal who commits suicide.

The evolutionary principle of natural selection—the survival of those best-fitted for the environment—would make us expect a rise in the suicide rate consistent with growth in population and increase in competitive activity.

More and more persons compete for fewer and fewer resources, hence the pressures on the individual increase dramatically. This has already been foreshadowed by comparisons of urban and rural health and crime statistics. Animal studies also indicate that overcrowding produces an increase in antisocial tendencies and aggressive behavior.

A further factor, mentioned previously, is the improvement in medical knowledge that enables a greater number of people to live a longer life-span. This has already given Western society a preponderance of aged persons, and the ratio will continue to increase for some time. As the aged are already one of the high-risk suicide groups, it seems logical to assume that the total number of suicides for almost all population groups will increase dramatically.

This has been illustrated with great realism in a number of films and books on the subject—one film going so far as to depict a suicide parlor where an easy death is administered in pleasant circumstances.

I cannot think of a more civilized approach to the problem. Suicide is a basic human right and should be an option always available to the individual. There is no need to assume any further curbs or checks on the process other than those already imposed on the prescription of addictive or lethal drugs, general medical treatment, or high-risk surgery.

All doctors are generally well-trained members of professional groups. Their province is the health of the individual. If life interferes with mental health, and the cessation of life is the only option (in the sense of the existential view that death may be good for the soul), then doctors are fully competent to prescribe suicide.

A prerequisite of course is major social change. Society will need to refocus on suicide and see it not as a problem but as a legitimate course of action. The political will to legislate for such change often lags behind the necessity, but in the end, social pressures force the issue.

An example is the decades-long soul-searching in Western countries over the use of birth control and family planning. Even today this has not been resolved, and there are countries in which they remain extralegal procedures. But in general, social pressure has forced reluctant legislatures to legitimize family planning programs.

Abortion, another emotionally weighted subject, is a strongly debated issue which remains a hot potato for any politician. But, as population growth gradually relegates the question almost to the level of non sequitur, legal barriers are falling one by one.

There is no need for alarm at what would seem to be a black picture of the future of the human race. All life, and not least in the case of homo sapiens, has a strong sense of self-preservation built into the genes. For humans, this is reflected in the structure of society—the accepted code of behavior that lubricates what would otherwise be the abrasive contact of individuals in the mass.

An example of this suicide countermeasure is the number of social agencies and nonprofessional groups that have come into being to help actively with counseling and other means of strengthening the individual's hold on life.

A few years ago my youngest brother, Marius, also a cardiac surgeon, and I stood at the bedside of one of our patients and watched him slowly suffocate from an advanced carcinoma of the lung.

The patient had been a good man, a man who had lived life well and dealt justly with his fellows. He had accepted his fate without complaint. While we stood there and watched him gasp for breath, he recognized us and was still able to put a ghost of a smile on his emaciated face. Conversation was impossible, yet in those sunken eyes there was a plea for help. There was only one effective form of help we could give him, and that was illegal.

When Marius and I walked away from his bed, shaken by our inability to comfort our patient, we turned to each other and vowed that each of us would help the other if we found ourselves in similar circumstances. We agreed that this could be done either with the administration of a fatal overdose (if the sufferer was incapable of helping himself) or by leaving within reach enough tablets so that the sufferer could take his own life.

I cannot speak for anyone else, but in my case it is not pain I fear. As a chronic arthritic, one learns to live with pain. What I fear most is becoming depersonalized—the ending of life that may come before death, the phase in which I would no longer be in control of my environment.

All my life I have held tight to my own concept of my world. It is a world that responds to my actions, that feeds back to me confirmation of my own being; a world that makes sense to me. Most people, I feel, have a similar relationship with their world.

Those are my requirements for life. Anything less is not living, and whatever it might be it is unacceptable. For that reason I wish to remain in control to the end, even if this should mean the bringing forward of that end.

Let me say that I have never agreed with those who claim that suffering ennobles.

The problem of human suffering has probably generated more discussion—much of it nonsense—than any other aspect of our daily condition. Philosophers, theologians, and wordsmiths take great care to classify suffering into acute, chronic, physical, and spiritual components—and then go on to dwell on the peculiarities of each.

Inevitably, the discussion will lead to the conclusion that suffering is an ennobling human experience.

Every time you hear or read that point of view you can be reasonably sure of one thing—that the person proposing it has not the faintest conception of suffering of any kind, least of all that involving physical pain. And physical pain is the kind most often encountered in the doctor-patient relationship.

Long acquaintance with human fallibility, most of it my own, has taught me never to be adamant on any subject. But if ever I were tempted to stick my neck out, it would be on this topic—and my first categorical statement would be that there is no nobility in pain, bravely borne or otherwise.

There is no nobility in the fishlike gasps of the patient trying to suck more air into bulging emphysematous lungs.

Neither is there nobility in the struggle of a patient who has both legs amputated at the hip to position himself on a bedpan.

I say that if suffering ennobles, then mankind would indeed be a noble breed, for is not suffering our normal lot?

Some schools of thought tell us that we are born

in terror and survive mentally only because we repress the memory, later to recall it when the going gets tough.

Certainly the lives of a vast number of the world's children are sagas of quiet desperation. According to figures released by the World Health Organization, of the 125 million infants that will be born this year, at least 12 million are unlikely to see their first birthday. Another 20 million may die before the age of five, and of those who survive, a percentage will be physical and mental cripples.

The great religions have always been concerned with the problem of human suffering, particularly with the paradox of a merciful God in a world that knows such suffering.

That paradox was resolved for me in my early training days as a resident doctor working in the United States. I met a man who made a great impression on me. He was Dr. Mel Williams of Richmond, Virginia, a lay preacher, a great scientist, and a good human being who once wrote a thesis on the power of prayer.

I remember chatting to him on his way to church one Sunday morning. I told him that my father had also been a preacher, and I asked him the theme of his sermon for the day.

He gave it in one sentence: "If God is good, there is no God; if God is bad, He is not God."

I puzzled over that for days until I realized what Mel meant. Human beings keep attributing human emotions to the Deity—a kind of reversal of the creation process, a re-creation of God in our own image.

Using human reasoning to arrive at the essence

of God was taken to the limits of logical absurdity by some schools of thought among the ancient Greeks, who conceived of God as perfection, or the perfect good. Logically, they said, such perfection can never be associated with imperfection, as that would make it less than perfect.

They reasoned that perfection was an absolute all-or-nothing state. Therefore, the totally perfect could only remain in the condition of total perfection as long as it did not partake of, come into contact with, or have any association with anything that was less than perfect.

Once agreed on that, the Greeks were forced to conclude that if God exists, and He could only exist in the perfect state, He cannot be aware of anything imperfect—and that includes the human race.

Hence God could not possibly know that the human race exists.

Such absurdities are of course the result of semantic problems—using language to construct analogies that are then resolved. The resolution is referred back to the original concept, giving the thinker the illusion that he has resolved the problem.

Ten

Therefore the Lord God sent him forth from the garden of Eden. . . . and He placed at the east of the garden of Eden the cherubim, and the flaming sword which turned every way, to keep the way to the tree of life.
—Genesis 3:23–24

The great religious myth of the expulsion of Adam and Eve from the Garden and their loss of status as immortal beings has a gripping fascination for all who read it. The account goes back thousands of years and is mirrored in many cultures. Yet it is only comparatively recently that scientists have discovered that the history of man's mortality is written in our body cells.

Another great literary myth, the Four Horsemen of the Apocalypse, symbolizes four agents of destruction—appearing to mankind as war, disease, famine, and death. They are represented in literature as eternally standing between man and immortality.

Laboratory work has virtually paralleled this view with the finding that the four barriers to eternal life for all living organisms—whether fish, flesh, fowl or plant—are disease, injury, famine, and aging.

And in spite of the tremendous triumphs of modern medicine, there is no evidence to show that from man's beginning to the present day these great leaps in knowledge and skill have increased the human life-span. Three of the great historical barriers have fallen, yet age remains like "the flaming sword which turned every way, to keep the way to the tree of life."

What *has* been achieved is a reduction of the likelihood of dying at an early age, thus increasing life expectancy because more individuals are reaching the unchanged upper age limit.

Dr. Leonard Hayflick, a leading authority on the cell biology of human aging who is now with the Bruce Lyon Memorial Research Laboratory in Oakland, California, has pointed out that if the two main causes of death in North America, namely heart disease and stroke, were successfully eliminated, only eighteen years of additional life could be expected.

If cancer, the third greatest cause of death, were eliminated, only about two years of additional life expectancy would result.

In the half century from 1900 to 1950, life expectancy in North America increased by a mere twenty years—owing mainly to the better understanding of hygiene, the rise in living standards, and the successful use of medicines to treat conditions that caused death before the age of sixty-five.

From 1900 to 1969 the gain in life expectancy at sixty-five and seventy-five years of age was only 2.9 and 2.2 years respectively.

A review of the literature makes it clear that of the four feared horsemen, but one is left—the "flaming sword" of senescence, or aging, that bars the way to the tree of life.

Let us have a look at what aging is all about. The human body is made up of three biological components: cells, such as the white corpuscles of the blood and those that line the gut, that divide and multiply throughout life; cells incapable of dividing and renewal, such as those in the brain; and noncellular material occurring as intercellular substance and collagen.

Aging is a gradual decline in the physiological efficiency of these components, resulting clinically in loss of vigor and in greater susceptibility to disease.

In an attempt to find out why this occurs and how it can be prevented, or at least postponed, scientists have evolved a new field of study—that of the cell biology of human aging. Such studies have now moved out of the field of eccentricity and have become an area of inquiry for the world's top biologists. Immortality is no longer a science-fiction word.

As a first approach to the study of aging, biologists decided that it would probably be more productive and simpler to start by examining the building blocks, or cells, of the organism.

This was achieved in two ways: through study of the behavior of cells in culture medium and through study of the behavior of cells serially transplanted into genetically similar recipients.

In 1961, while studying a cell culture, Dr. Hayflick and his colleagues made a significant discovery.

They found when particular cells were placed in a culture medium, in this case the fibroblasts from a human embryo, the cells underwent a finite number of doublings and then died. The Hayflick study demonstrated that even if these cells were grown under optimal conditions, death followed after fifty doublings.

The conclusion was that the death of these cells was not due to an environmental inadequacy but to some inherent property of the cells themselves—in other words, we carry our own death warrants written in our cell structure.

This was further substantiated by taking cells that had undergone a number of divisions, or doublings, and freezing them. The lowered temperature arrested biological activity. Various stages of cell division were selected as the freezing points, and samples were stored at reduced temperatures for varying lengths of time. The cells were then reconstituted and allowed to divide further in a culture medium.

They went right ahead and doubled up as before—but only to the allotted fifty times. In other words, cells arrested at 10 doublings continued through another 40 doublings before dying, while cells arrested at 45 doublings added only another 5 doublings before death. This was the case no matter how the length of the freezing time was varied.

The study demonstrated that normal human embryo fibroblasts live in a culture medium for a fixed number of reproductive cycles before they die. Research workers reasoned that if this was a manifestation of senescence at the cellular level, it could be confirmed experimentally by testing cells from various human age-groups.

It should follow logically that cells taken from an adult rather than an embryo would not be able to divide fifty times because a certain amount of aging had already taken place.

This proved to be the case. Normal human adult fibroblasts were allowed to divide in a culture medium. Their total number of doublings was significantly less than those of the embryo cells. The finding indicates an inverse relation between the age of the human donor and the *in vitro* (outside the body) proliferation capacity of these cells.

Another avenue of research was the phenomenon of progeria, or precocious aging, a condition in which the patient at the age of ten years shows physical signs of aging normally found in a person of seventy years.

Fibroblasts were cultured from patients suffering from progeria to see to what extent the cells would multiply and survive. It was predicted that their life-span would be measurably shortened.

The assumption was correct. Cells from progeriatric patients divided from 2 to 10 times, where the normal values were between 20 and 40.

The next step was to demonstrate that what happened *in vitro* also happened *in vivo* (in the body). To do this, cells were labeled so that they could be identified. The labeled cells were transplanted from one genetically identical host to another as soon as the donor approached old age.

Such cells did not survive beyond their programmed limit. The injury of transplantation seemed to have little effect, and survival appeared related only to the age of the grafted cells.

There is wide variation in the life-span of various species. To take extreme pairing: The mayfly lives only a few hours; an elephant lives for many decades.

Experiments were carried out to see if there was any correlation between the population doubling of cultured normal fibroblasts and the mean maximum life-span of the species. The findings were not conclusive, but a trend showed.

For example, normal embryo fibroblasts from a tortoise—with a life-span of some 150 years—were grown in culture media and achieved doublings of up to 125. In contrast, normal embryo fibroblasts from a mouse with a life-span of 2.5 years showed between 14 and 28 doublings.

The experimental evidence presented up to this point suggests the strong possibility of a direct relationship between the ability of cells to divide and the process of aging. The conclusion is almost inescapable that—with one startling exception—all cells in the end face the fourth horseman.

The exception is a disturbing one. In cell culture laboratories throughout the world, cancer cells, taken in 1952 from human carcinoma at the mouth of the womb, have continued to flourish through innumerable doublings even to this day.

The discovery of "immortal cells" presented a major headache to biologists interested in senescence, until it became clear that such cells were abnormal, whereas cells that showed a fixed number of doublings were normal.

Abnormality in the immortal cells could be due either to a morphological deviation in the nucleus and chromosomes (genetic material) when compared to the genetic material of the cells from which they were originally derived, or there could be a distinct difference in the way the genetic material of the immortal cells expressed itself when compared to the genetic expression of the cells from which they arose.

This can be shown by taking a mortal cell and

infecting it with a cancer virus. The infection brings about a fusion of the genetic material of the virus and that of the cell, making the genetic material abnormal. The immediate result is that the cell becomes immortal.

Up to this point, one is almost forced to conclude that human senescence is due to one or more important cell population losing the ability to divide and replenish. Further experimental work has shown that this is only part of the aging process. Major functional changes take place in normal human cells grown *in vitro* and are expressed well before the cells lose their capacity to replicate.

It is therefore important to recognize that the cessation of the ability of the cell to divide is only one functional deterioration whose genetic basis may be similar to that known to occur in nondividing cells, such as those of the brain and muscle.

Dr. Hayflick summed this up by saying that it was not his contention that age changes result necessarily from loss of cell division capacity, but simply from loss of function in any class of cells. Function loss may be measured as reduced division capacity, or any number of myriad other functional deteriorations characteristic of aging cells.

This physiological decay of the cells probably has a common denominator in that loss of population-doubling potential *in vitro* may have the same basis as the loss of other cell functions characteristic of nondividing cells. It is logical to assume that if we understand the mechanism by which cultured normal cells lose their capacity to divide, this could also provide an insight into the causes of deterioration in the functional properties that are characteristic of nondividing cells and that may be even more direct causes of biological aging.

If the loss of proliferation capacity in a cell population is an expression of aging (which appears to be the case on evidence), then it is important to locate and understand the mechanism that controls this finite repetitive capacity in order to manipulate it in an attempt to increase man's life-span.

Through a very ingenious experiment, Hayflick and his colleagues proved that the proliferation mechanism is genetically controlled. The fourth horseman, the flaming sword that forbids a return to Eden, is located in the nucleus of the cell.

They showed this by taking cultured cells and treating them with a chemical called Cytochalasin B. This caused the cell to extrude its nucleus, and by centrifugation, millions of cells without nuclei (without genetic information) were obtained.

These anucleated cells were called cytoplasts, and they remained alive for several days. Using a special technique, the genetic information of old cells was introduced into young cytoplasts while nuclei of young cells were introduced into old cytoplasts.

This produced young cells with old genetic information and old cells with young genetic information.

Studies of the remaining population doublings showed that young cells with old genetic information had less replication power than old cells with young nuclei. The conclusion was that the life-span of man is fixed and that it is genetically programmed into his cell structure.

To understand more fully the genetic basis of aging, what is required is a clearer grasp of the fundamentals of genetic control of the cells themselves. It has been demonstrated experimentally that insertion of the nucleus of an intestinal cell of a tadpole into the anucleated ovum of a frog will produce a frog identical to the tadpole from which the nucleus was taken.

A similar result can be obtained by using the nuclei of other cells of the body, for example, skin or liver cells. This means that every cell in the body probably contains all the genetic information necessary to reproduce another individual identical to the donor.

The question arises why, under certain circumstances, only a very small proportion of the vast store of available knowledge is used. Why, for example, do liver cells produce only the proteins necessary for liver function and muscle cells only the proteins necessary for muscle function, when any single cell has enough genetic information to rebuild the entire organism?

Although it is not clearly understood, it appears that in the case of the liver cell, only the information necessary to make the specific proteins for liver function are transmitted to the factory or cytoplasm of the cell, and similarly for muscle cells. Once a cell has differentiated to carry out a specific function, only a small portion of the genetic information is used from then onward.

Like individual members of the orchestra, each cell plays its own complementary music even though capable of reproducing the whole symphony. If aging is thus an inability of the cell to use genetic information correctly, we may get a better understanding of what goes wrong if we can find out what induces a particular cell to play the part of the oboe rather than the flute.

It stretches the imagination to reflect that all the cell types in the human body arise from one fertilized cell—the ovum, or egg.

This is made possible as a result of two processes: cell division, which allows cells to multiply; and a series of "one-way" differentiation processes, which cause cells to take up different functions. The ovum, once fertilized, starts dividing to form two daughter cells and then dividing again to form 4, 8, 16, 32, and so on. The second process, that of differentiation, sets in at about the 32-cell stage. Until this point all the cells look the same and react the same. From here on they look different and are different from each other in terms of their manufacture of protein and enzymes.

Cell differentiation is the result of the activation of certain genes while others are restrained, thus preventing the formation of unwanted proteins. The mechanism of repression is almost certainly chemically controlled and will one day be understood.

In 1977, a South African Medical Research Council Unit in the Department of Medical Biochemistry at the University of Stellenbosch Medical School reported an interesting research achievement.

These investigators took a culture of cells removed from a mouse embryo that closely resembled fibroblasts (the cells that form scar tissue). The culture was treated with a chemical called 5-Azacytidine, and it was found that the cells reacted by differentiating into muscle cells. Not only did they stand up to examination under the microscope, they also contracted under chemical stimulation in the same way as did muscle cells.

Similar results have been achieved with the use of other chemical compounds. But how does this throw light on the problem of aging?

It is very likely that aging is the end result of differentiation. It represents a failure to divide or a failure to continue accurately to make the functional cell proteins. If this is so, then the most likely control agent is chemical—superimposed on the differentiation program of each cell as it occurs in each cell except the germ cell.

In other words, aging may represent a further repression of genes, which is chemically controlled. As this form of control is more clearly understood and the genetic messages unraveled, the possibility of the control of aging will become a reality.

But, until such time as biologists have discovered the exact makeup of this elixir of life, we will have to be satisfied with cruder means of increasing the life-span. One way would be to leave this world physiologically while remaining here physically, as do animals who hibernate in the winter and "return" to life in the summer.

However, the search for immortality demands more than a mere escape for the space of a winter. Suspended animation, achieved by deep-freezing as opposed to hibernation, has been mooted. Theoretically, this process will stop all physiological body activities.

The snag, as highlighted by Hayflick's work, is that this will not increase man's active life but merely his physical existence—since aging will continue from where it left off when the body was frozen.

It has been argued that deep-freezing could be of great help in keeping human beings preserved alive until such time as the disease from which they are dying can be cured.

The idea had always struck me as frivolous until by chance I came across Gordon R. Taylor's *Biological Time Bomb*. Here was a whole new world of people with sublime faith in the prospect of icing their way into eternity.

In the United States a number of organizations have been formed to push ahead with experimental work in cryogenics. Examples are the Life Extension Society of Washington, the Immortality Research and Complication Association, and the Anabiosis and Longevity Institute of New York.

A number of people have paid large sums of money to ensure that at death, their bodies will be preserved by freezing in the belief that the techniques of successful revival will eventually be developed.

I was amazed to learn that in California in 1967 a retired professor of psychology, Dr. James H. Bedford, set aside more than four thousand dollars for this purpose before he died of cancer at the age of seventy-three.

The technology governing the process is reasonably simple. Immediately after his death, Dr. Bedford was injected with heparin, a substance that prevents clotting of the blood. His chest was then opened and his heart massaged in order to supply his brain with oxygenated blood until such time as his body could be connected to a heart-lung machine.

Once on the machine, his temperature was progressively lowered to 8°C by packing ice around the body. At this point, most of the blood was withdrawn and replaced with a solution of salt plus a solvent known as DMSO (Dimethyl Sulfoxide).

The temperature of the body was lowered a further 87 degrees to −79°C and was then flown to Phoenix, Arizona, for storage in liquid oxygen at −190°C.

It all sounds pretty straightforward. Unfortunately, the freezing of organs and whole bodies is not that easy. Damage occurs in tissues kept at low temperatures for long periods, and further damage takes place when the temperature is raised again.

This is due, in part, to the physical changes that take place in liquids at low temperatures, inducing stresses in surrounding tissue. To take one aspect, as water in the cells freezes, the concentration of salts builds up until it reaches a damaging level. In addition, the change in volume creates ice crystals that puncture the cell wall.

Were it not for the fact that any researcher learns early to use the word *impossible* with caution, most scientists would be tempted to place such work in the realm of the ridiculous.

Only a few years ago, who would have thought that mammalian cells such as blood cells, spermatozoa, fibroblasts—for that matter, any tissues capable of conversion into single cell form—could be stored at low temperatures for years?

Yet it has been shown that a suspension of the cells in nutrient solution mixed with DMSO can be cooled to −190°C and then stored. When required, the cells can be thawed and washed, and full physiological function is restored.

Progress has also been made in the length of storage of organs. Today, kidneys are removed on one continent, stored and transported to another continent, and transplanted successfully with immediate function. In my own laboratories, it has been demonstrated that a heart can be taken from an animal, stored without being perfused with blood for twenty-four hours, and transplanted into another animal to give sufficient immediate function to keep it alive.

If successful storage of human beings by deep freezing one day becomes a reality, there will obviously be far-reaching social and economic problems. How, for example, would the deep-freeze person's will be handled? Would such a person be subject to estate taxes? Would he or she still have a vote? Would such persons be allowed to marry their great-great-grandchildren (there is no law against it now)? The possibilities for social, legal, and ethical tangles are enormous.

Until such time as we can outwit the fourth horseman and prevent senescence and death in the cell, it seems that organ transplantation remains the partial answer to longevity. By this process, such components as the kidney, the heart, the bone marrow, and to a lesser extent the liver, provide a way in which old, worn-out, or diseased organs can be replaced by young healthy ones.

Further, as soon as we conquer the problem of making nerve connections that give the immediate function we have achieved with blood vessels, then transplantation of body parts that depend on nerve function, such as the limbs and the brain, will be within the realm of possibility.

Research in electronics makes possible many scenarios once regarded as figments of the imagination. Metal implants as skeletal assists have been in use for decades. Total hip replacement is now a reality. Now comes the possibility of self-organizing electronic structures existing at the molecular level.

Most people have heard of the microchip revolution which has created the minicomputers or microprocessors—tiny slivers of material containing thousands of switching circuits and capable of carrying out a number of functions more quickly and cheaply than ever thought possible.

The next step is the superchip, smaller than the naked eye can see, built at the molecular level and packed with millions—as opposed to mere thousands in the microchip—of transistors. They have already been predicted by the British theoretical physicist, Dr. John Barker, who has devised a theoretical framework for understanding such phenomena.

His work indicates that when components reach a degree of miniaturization where they are no bigger than individual molecules, they undergo dramatic physical changes. Suddenly they are no longer discrete electronic components in the normal sense of the word, but they become dependent on their neighbors and spontaneously form couplings between each other.

Dr. Barker says the possibility exists that such devices could organize themselves in ways comparable to that of living organisms. For example, they could "heal" a damaged component and even learn to program themselves.

This poses a future where such atomic-scale chips would become spare parts for man, literally used as plug-in additions or improvements to the body to bypass or correct faulty functioning. The auditory nerve could be "wired" to overcome deafness, eye damage could be bypassed with modular components, and it might even be possible to replace damaged brain areas with a bio-chip. The possibilities are limited only by the imagination.

At present there is ample evidence to indicate that man's search for immortality is gaining ground. The thought is disturbing. Although long-term survival may benefit the individual, there is cause to think that it would be of great harm to the species as a whole.

Senescence and death are an evolutionary necessity. The built-in cell program in each species allows enough time, whether measured in hours or years, for each individual in its lifetime to mature, adapt to its short-term environment, and reproduce.

If the individual cannot cope with the environment, he will not reproduce, and his genes will die with him. On a large enough scale this can wipe out a whole species. The fossil record of the earth shows that this has happened many times in the past. Evolution is a hard taskmaker and only the successful survive.

Those who cope with the changing environment do so because of some evolutionary change in their genes, some slight quirk or mutation which when reproduced enables the offspring to survive. Hence, in an environment of fast-moving predators, the slightly faster rabbit will live to pass on his athletic genes to his offspring while his slothful neighbor will never know what hit him.

If an individual *should* live forever, he eventually would become an evolutionary contradiction, an organism carrying unchanging genes unable to adapt to the changing environment. Apart from overpopulation, which could in itself cause major changes in the environment, the species could quickly become obsolete.

Sir George Pickering expressed this so aptly when he said, "Insofar as man is an improvement of monkeys, this is due to death. A new species, for better or for worse, can only start with a new life."

It is appropriate that I end my reflections on death and dying with a nod to the cell biologists and other researchers who are working to arrest the onslaught of aging.

A half century ago, A. S. Warden wrote, "We live but to create a new machine of a little later model than our own, a new life machine that in some ineffable way can help along the great process of evolution of the species somehow more efficiently than we could do if we were immortal."

Who knows what sort of new life machine will emerge as a result of new discoveries in genetic engineering and cell biology. Perhaps in years to come there will be no need to plea for a saner attitude toward those individuals who would be better off if their life were to cease.

For the present, however, there is no question that each of us is mortal and that death is an essential part of life. It is thus the duty of society to create an environment in which every individual will be able to live a good life—and to die a good death.

.

—Appendix—

The Oath of Hippocrates

How often we hear reference to the Oath of Hippocrates in relation to the ethics of medicine and to the accepted standards of a physician's practice. What is this time-honored oath?

In reality, the Oath of Hippocrates is a mythological canon which stemmed from Judeo-Christian ideals. Dr. Markley H. Boyer of the Harvard School of Public Health says, "Hippocrates is what we should be. His image serves as a spiritual guide by which we discharge our duties to ourselves, our colleagues, and our patients."

As mentioned in this volume, the oath is no longer generally accepted by practitioners who emerge from a different culture and religious background. On the other hand, it is part of medical history and must be respected for providing the model for our forefathers in the medical profession.

Here is how the most recent, accepted, version reads:

"I swear by Apollo, the physician, and Asclepius and Health and All-Heal and all the gods and goddesses that, according to my ability and judgment, I will keep this oath and stipulation:

"To reckon him who taught me this art equally dear to me as my parents, to share my substance with him and relieve his necessities if required; to regard his offspring as on the same footing with my own brothers, and to teach them this art if they should wish to learn it, without fee or stipulation, and that by precept, lecture and every other mode of instruction, I will impart a knowledge of the art to my own sons and to those of my teachers, and to disciples bound by a stipulation and oath, according to the law of medicine, but to none others.

"I will follow that method of treatment which, according to my ability and judgment, I consider for the benefit of my patients, and abstain from whatever is deleterious and mischievous. I will give no deadly medicine to anyone if asked, nor suggest any such counsel; furthermore, I will not give to a woman an instrument to produce abortion.

"With purity and with holiness I will pass my life and practice my art. I will not cut a person who is suffering with a stone, but will leave this to be done by practitioners of this work. Into whatever houses I enter I will go into them for the benefit of the sick and will abstain from every voluntary act of mischief and corruption; and further from the seduction of females or males, bond or free.

"Whatever, in connection with my professional

practice, or not in connection with it, I may see or hear in the lives of men which ought not to be spoken abroad I will not divulge, as reckoning that all such should be kept secret.

"While I continue to keep this oath unviolated may it be granted to me to enjoy life and the practice of the art, respected by all men at all times but should I trespass and violate this oath, may the reverse be my lot."

Model State Law for Determination of Death

A giant step has been taken in the legal consideration of when an individual should be considered dead. In the United States, the American Medical Association has urged the individual state legislatures to adopt a model law—the result of currently accepted medical practice and of many years of ethical, legal, and civic debate.

The model law reads as follows (comments are those of the AMA):

"*Section 1.* An individual who has sustained either (1) irreversible cessation of circulatory and respiratory functions, or (2) irreversible cessation of all functions of the entire brain, shall be considered dead. A determination of death shall be made in accordance with accepted medical standards.

["COMMENT: This section is intended to provide a comprehensive statement for determining death in all situations, by clarifying and codifying the common law in this regard. The two bases set forth in the statute are the only medically accepted bases for determining death, and the statute is therefore all inclusive. 'All functions' of the brain means that purposeful activity of the brain, as distinguished from random activity in the brain, has ceased. 'Entire brain' includes both the brain stem and the neocortex and is meant to distinguish the concept of neocortical death, which is not a valid medical basis for determining death.

"It is recognized that physicians may determine death. It is also recognized that in some jurisdictions non-physicians (i.e. coroners) are empowered to determine death. It is the intent of this bill to recognize that under accepted medical standards a determination of death based on irreversible cessation of brain function may be made only by a physician.]

"*Section 2.* A physician or any other person authorized by law to determine death who makes such determination in accordance with Section 1 is not liable for damages in any civil action or subject to prosecution in any criminal proceeding for his acts or the acts of others based on that determination.

"*Section 3.* Any person who acts in good faith in reliance on a determination of death is not liable for damages in any civil action or subject to prosecution in any criminal proceeding for his act.

["COMMENT: While Section 1 is intended to remove legal impediments relating to a declaration of death based on medically accepted principles, Sections 2 and 3 are intended to remove inhibitions from making a declaration of death based on either of the two standards and also to remove inhibitions of hospital personnel from carrying out the direction of a physician in this regard by removing the threat of liability.

These Sections do not absolve from liability a person who acts negligently or contrary to accepted medical standards.]

"*Section 4.* If any provision of this Act is held by a court to be invalid such invalidity shall not affect the remaining provisions of the Act, and to this end the provisions of this Act are hereby declared to be severable."

Index

143